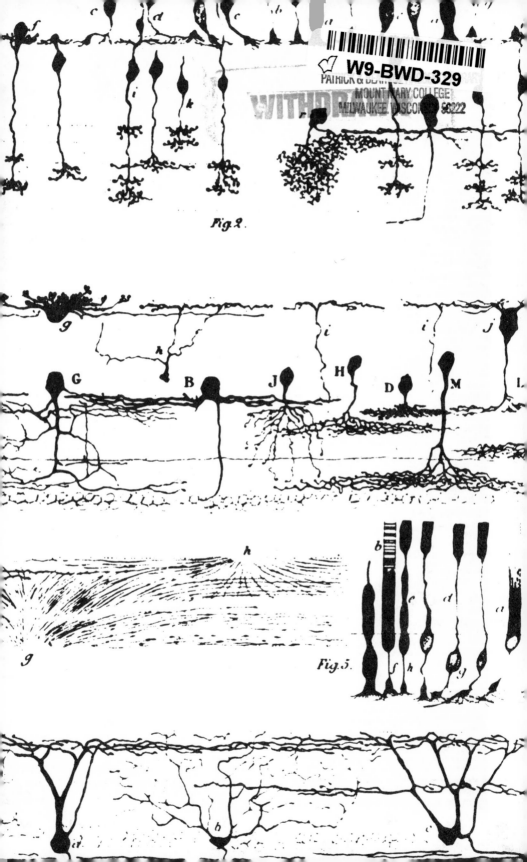

Fig. 2.

Fig. 5.

DISCOVERING THE

BRAIN

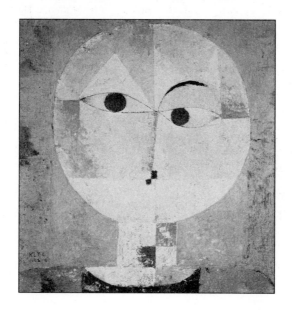

Sandra Ackerman
for the
INSTITUTE OF MEDICINE
NATIONAL ACADEMY OF SCIENCES

NATIONAL ACADEMY PRESS
Washington, D.C. 1992

National Academy Press • 2101 Constitution Avenue, N.W. • Washington, D.C. 20418

This publication is based on presentations at a July 1990 symposium organized by the Institute of Medicine and held in Washington, D.C., to initiate the Decade of the Brain.

The Institute of Medicine was chartered in 1970 by the National Academy of Sciences to enlist distinguished members of appropriate professions in the examination of policy matters pertaining to the health of the public. In this, the Institute acts both under the Academy's 1863 congressional charter responsibility to be an adviser to the federal government and its own initiative in identifying issues of medical care, research, and education.

This project was supported by the National Institute of Mental Health under contract number 278-90-0006(OD).

This book is printed with soy ink on acid-free recycled stock.

Library of Congress Cataloging-in-Publication Data
Discovering the brain / Sandra Ackerman for the Institute
  of Medicine
      p. cm.
  "Based on presentations at a July 1990 symposium organized by the
Institute of Medicine and held in Washington, D.C."—T.p. verso.
  "This project was supported by the National Institute of Mental
Health under contract number 278-90-0006 (OD)"—T.p. verso.
  Includes bibliographical references and index.
  ISBN 0-309-04529-0
  1. Brain. 2. Neurology. 3. Neurobiology. 4. United States.
Joint Resolution to Designate the Decade Beginning January 1, 1990,
as the "Decade of the Brain"—Congresses. I. Institute of Medicine
(U.S.) II. National Institute of Mental Health (U.S.) III. Title.
  [DNLM: 1. Brain. WL 300 A182d 1990]
QP376.A23 1992
612.8'2—dc20
DNLM/DLC
for Library of Congress   92-1231
                                                              CIP

Printed in the United States of America

The serpent has been a symbol of long life, healing, and knowledge among almost all cultures and religions since the beginning of recorded history. The image adopted as a logotype by the Institute of Medicine is based on a relief carving from ancient Greece, now held by the Staatlichemuseen in Berlin.

Cover: Paul Klee. *Senecio (Baldgreis).* 1922. Oil on canvas. Collection Öffentliche Kunstsammlung, Basel, Switzerland.

Foreword

The brain is the last and grandest biological frontier, the most complex thing we have yet discovered in our universe. It contains hundreds of billions of cells interlinked through trillions of connections. The brain boggles the mind.

The diseases that disrupt brain function are among the most painful and destructive we know—Alzheimer's disease, schizophrenia, Huntington's disease, and others. They invade the mind, tearing at the fabric of family life and shattering the attributes that make us most human. These diseases are the enemy; neuroscientists are fighters on the front lines. Their weapons are new ideas, tested by experimentation. The revolution in modern biology has supplied science with a formidable armamentarium, well stocked with purchases made using federal dollars.

The health of neuroscience today rests firmly on this foundation of public investment. Since World War II, our nation has consistently supported biomedical research, creating the most robust research enterprise the world has ever seen. That success, evidenced by the prizes and international recognition accorded American scientists, has depended on champions within government.

Silvio Conte was one such champion, a true friend of science. He passionately believed biomedical research could stop the ravages of incurable disease. Year after year, he supported such research in Congress. One of his last legislative acts was to shepherd a congressional resolution declaring the 1990s the "Decade of the Brain" through the congressional process, resulting in the official proclamation by President Bush in July 1989.

This book arose out of a July 1990 symposium organized by the Institute of Medicine to initiate the Decade of the Brain, the first installment in what will certainly develop into many decades of fruitful research. Rep. Conte attended the IOM symposium near the end of his public career. He died in office later that year. He will be sorely missed, especially by those who commit their lives to science. This book is dedicated to him.

The symposium was a political event with a scientific purpose. Scientists reviewed the state of their knowledge in the presence of policymakers, covering topics that ranged from the molecular events underlying transmission of nerve impulses to the biology of perception and consciousness. Sandra Ackerman is to be congratulated on her clear distillation of themes from the symposium into this book, which introduces neuroscience to those who may be approaching it for the first time. It serves as a clear overview of neuroscience in the early 1990s, as the molecular tools developed over the past three decades are becoming sufficiently powerful to allow us to navigate through an intellectual terrain as vast as the human brain.

James D. Watson
Director, Cold Spring Harbor Laboratory, and
Director, National Center for Human
    Genome Research
National Institutes of Health

Contents

DISCOVERING THE

BRAIN

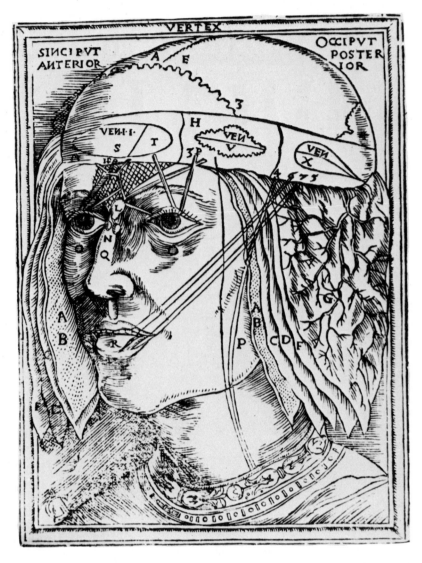

FIGURE 1.1. The earliest efforts to explore the brain arose from the same deep curiosity that draws researchers into neuroscience today. This Dutch woodcut from J. Dryander's *Anatomie* (1537) shows that the brain was already understood at this time as a structure composed of diverse parts. The woodcut identifies divisions between a frontal ("sinciput, anterior") and rear ("occipital, posterior") portion of the brain, and between lobes at the sides; these divisions still serve as landmarks for students of neuroanatomy. At the right, the letters A, B, C, D, F, and G distinguish the six layers of the cerebral cortex; in this century, observations down to the level of single cells make it possible to sort out the distinct functions of each of these layers. Source: The National Library of Medicine.

1

The Promise of Neuroscience

The demands of everyday life leave little time or reason to think about how we do what we do. Yet at any given moment innumerable and imperceptible transactions are occurring within the central nervous system—when we wake in the morning and shake off the impressions of a dream; when we go out for a walk, recognize a friend, and cross the street to say hello. The workings of the nervous system convey perceptions and states of mind that we can recognize and put a name to, and they make it possible for us to exchange signals—through language and in other forms—with other beings like ourselves. This same complex system even lets us screen out information, filtering our perceptions to highlight only what is different or noteworthy at the moment.

The brain is active throughout every day, even as we sleep, but we rarely, if ever, stop to consider that our thoughts, actions, and perceptions are the outcome of several trillion signals exchanged among nerve cells. The brain is such an efficient processor of information that most of the time we do not realize the magnitude of its task. Usually only a disruption of the nervous system—through disease or injury or inherited predisposition—calls our attention to the brain's myriad functions.

For instance, what is the "movement center" in the brain that is thought to degenerate in Parkinson's disease? How can chemical compounds in brain cells influence the emotions we feel? Why does injury at a particular site on the head leave some patients unable to recognize an arm or a leg as part of their own body? Neuroscience is the field of study that endeavors to make sense of such diverse questions; at the same time, it points the way toward the effective treatment of dysfunctions. The exchange of information among a half-dozen branches of science and the clinical practice of mental health have shaped a new scientific approach to the study of the brain.

The fruitfulness of this approach reaches far beyond the health care and research professions into most people's everyday lives. The research itself has a wide range of applications, from alleviating many hundreds of nervous and mental diseases to enriching the lives of the healthy. Key policymakers supported this research. The United States Congress in 1989 passed a resolution sponsored by Congressman Silvio Conte declaring the 1990s to be the Decade of the Brain. Following the official proclamation by President George Bush, the 1990 symposium on the Decade of the Brain attracted the participation of First Lady Barbara Bush, Secretary of Health and Human Services Louis W. Sullivan, Science Adviser to the President D. Allan Bromley, Congressman Conte, Senator Pete V. Domenici, and others.

At the beginning of the 1990s, neuroscience combines mature theory, lively new possibilities for investigation, and technology that can yield information unheard of even a few years ago: the genetic markers for an inherited predisposition toward some mental disorder, or the intimate structure, down to the individual molecules, of a receptor in the brain for a particular chemical compound, or medical images that convey the flow of energy in different areas while the brain manages such tasks as reading and thinking. The end of the decade may see the picture more richly detailed in some areas and changed almost beyond recognition in others.

In July 1990, a symposium brought scientists from all over the world to the National Academy of Sciences in Washington, D.C., to discuss the state of the field. Dominick Purpura, professor of neuroscience and vice president for medical affairs at Albert Einstein College of Medicine, Yeshiva University, addressed the gathering on the subject of "the brain's new science." He posed three basic questions: What is this endeavor known as the brain's new science? What makes it new? And what can it do for humankind?

APPROACHING THE BRAIN FROM ALL ANGLES

Neuroscience, in Purpura's thinking, is not a discipline—a statement that may come as a mild shock to some of its practitioners. Neuroscience is, rather, a *way to approach* specific questions about the structure and function of the human brain, whether in healthy development or when afflicted with injury or disease. Neuroscientific investigation may require the hands-on familiarity of neuroanatomy and physiology, the biochemical framework of neuroimmunology, or the specialized calculations of genetics; it may call for the bright scans of neural images that must be "read" with an eye for subtle changes, or the observation of full-scale behavior, as studied in neuropsychology; it can involve the advanced mathematics of the computational sciences and the intricate cellular workings of molecular biology. Purpura imagines all these approaches to be like the colors of a rainbow, spread out by a prism. Neuroscience represents the sum of these approaches, the white light by which we can see and understand.

Study of the brain can be more illuminating, of course, when it takes in the larger physical system of which it is a part. With all its intricate and powerful circuitry, the brain does not work in isolation. It shares in the circulation of the blood with the rest of the body; its cells require oxygen and nutrients and rely on the body's processes for fighting infection and for repair. Clearly, the physical state of the body can impinge on the brain in good health or in a great number of diseases or disorders that disrupt behavior or hobble the ability to think or feel. And everyone is familiar, if only by hearsay, with the "psychosomatic" headache or back pain that gives physical expression to something experienced in the mind; this is the brain-body influence working in the opposite direction. Enoch Gordis, director of the National Institute on Alcohol Abuse and Alcoholism, offers another example of this interrelationship. Understanding the role of the liver and kidneys in handling drugs and toxins may be crucial for treating substance abuse and addictions—among the most vexing problems in public health today.

Over the years many nonscientists, too, have contributed to neuroscientific knowledge in the role of research subjects, whether in the clinical setting of the neurologist's office or as volunteers performing a cognitive task in the psychology laboratory. The two-way channel of information continues to expand: findings from the laboratory lead toward sharper criteria for diagnosing mental disorders and more effective methods for treating them, and in turn the clinician's increasingly acute skills of diagnosis and observation supply the research scientist with more precise data for study in the lab.

The data under examination in such laboratories often come in forms that would have been unimaginable a decade or two ago. But the research itself proceeds from the same basic ideas that guided the very first investigations in neuroscience. Essential to an understanding of the nervous system is the notion that the body experiences signals, or nerve impulses, both from the outside environment and from its own inner functioning; to keep these numerous signals from producing a chaos of sensation, the body organizes them into patterns. The nervous system, particularly the brain, carries out this task, not only organizing but also translating the signals into information the body can use—to activate a group of muscles, quicken the heartbeat, or recall the sight of a familiar face.

More recently, scientists have come up with the idea of a *chain* of signals, each with its unique function in the series. First are the signals that pass from one whole nerve cell to another by means of electrical impulses or the chemical compounds known as neurotransmitters. Next come the "second messengers," which broadcast a signal within one nerve cell; in response, a group of enzymes, the protein kinases, may convert another compound in the cell from its inactive state to an active one. The switched-on substance, in turn, acts in conjunction with a possible "third messenger," a substrate that brings its own chemical factors into the formula. However long the chain of processes may appear, each link adds something necessary and irreplaceable—whether by fine-tuning the signal or by helping to spread it throughout a region.

A scientific principle that has brought together some diverse findings in neuroscience is "parsimony in nature." Simply put, this is the idea that natural processes or systems first observed in one context, for which they appear beautifully fitted, tend to turn up again in other contexts, sometimes filling other functions—to which they seem equally well suited. The neurotransmitters illustrate this notion: for instance, norepinephrine dilates the blood vessels in muscle tissue but causes the opposite effect, constriction, in the blood vessels of the skin. Thus it appears that nature has conserved the one transmitter and thriftily made it over to another use by having it interact with different receptor sites in the two contexts. Another striking instance of this principle is found in certain physical changes in the nervous system that accompany learning in very simple animals. In the marine snail *Aplysia*, a newly learned behavior is associated with the growth of signal-transmitting elements from its nerve cells. At the time of this new growth, the levels of cell-adhesion proteins drop briefly but significantly. This change in levels suggests to researchers that the proteins may actually serve to inhibit such extra growth much of the time, when learning is *not* taking place in the animal. By contrast, outside the brain, cell-adhesion proteins are much better known for their crucial role in the immune system, where they aid in the attachment of disease-fighting antibodies. In yet another context, cell-adhesion proteins may play a still different role in the development of a baby's brain, by guiding the migration of nerve cells to the six-layered cerebral cortex that covers most of the brain like the bark of a tree.

"When neuroscience works well, it begins to unify data," says Dominick Purpura. Such indeed was the effect of a recent feat in the research world: the mapping of the precise connections in the basal ganglia, deep inside the brain. In primates, this region was known in relatively little detail until recently. The basal ganglia are important for the control of movement, for which they receive signals from the cerebral cortex; electrical recordings show both these areas to be active a fraction of a second before a movement takes place. To map the pathways of these nerve signals has called for a solid foundation of anatomy, highly refined techniques for the selective staining of particular cells, and close studies of signal-carrying agents such as messenger RNA. With the pathways identified, both for nerve impulses that inhibit movement and for those that initiate it, researchers can begin to build new explanations of what goes wrong in neurological diseases that lead to disorders of movement, such as Parkinson's and early-stage Huntington's disease. They may be in a better position, too, to explain less well known diseases such as hemiballism, in which the patient involuntarily undergoes repeated, purposeless movements of the arm or leg that resemble jumping or throwing a ball.

Stronger hypotheses about the mechanism of a disease can point the way toward more effective treatment and new possibilities for a cure. In highly complex disorders of the brain, in which many factors—genetic, environmental, epidemiological, even social and psychological—play a part, broadly based hypotheses are exceedingly useful. As Purpura says, "The problem here is to study how the system works, and that's what makes it neuroscience—not whether one is using molecular biology, electrophysiology, or any other particular aspect."

WHAT MAKES THIS SCIENCE NEW?

Because neuroscience is so broadly based, drawing on research from many points across the scientific landscape, it is not easy to sort out the elements that make this science of the brain "new." The fact is that neuroscience has not sprung from a revolutionary theory or a startling reversal of all that was known before; rather, the approach builds on a set of principles that, in scientific parlance, are unlikely to be proved untrue. (This cautious phrasing means that the principles have held up in rigorous testing so far, in a great variety of settings; but scientists stop short of guaranteeing them against future refinements or corrections, since a willingness to test—rather than to keep faith—is a hallmark of science.) One such principle is the current understanding that nerve cells can be excited by both electrical and chemical signals and that both types of signals act by altering the flow of ions (positively or negatively charged particles) into or out of the cell. Another principle holds that the development of the brain allows room for shaping by the environment (everything from nutrition and the family setting to incidence of disease) and that the two shaping forces, environmental and genetic, act on each other in an intricate weave, creating in every person's head a pattern of connections that is unique and yet recognizable within the standard form.

Is there something special about the 1990s that makes this the Decade of the Brain? Enoch Gordis answers this question with an emphatic "yes": the research that is possible, or is already taking place, represents not just an extension of earlier efforts but a qualitative change. From a base of knowledge about the brain in general, neuroscience is now making the first exploratory inroads into the features that characterize us as human: the ability to create and to calculate, to empathize, to recall and plan, and perhaps even to develop illnesses that are uniquely human, such as schizophrenia or the problems of substance abuse.

Advances in technology offer opportunities to examine the human brain not as inert anatomical matter but in its living, functional state. (For a survey of these methods, see Chapter 3.) Using positron emission tomography (PET), researchers and clinicians can trace changes in activity from one region of the brain to another as the individual carries out a mental task (for instance, recognizing the written form of words and sorting them into categories). More than that: because the imaging computer receives and coordinates an enormous amount of information from a single scan, it is possible to produce a series of images—almost like a dissection—with each image representing a different layer of functioning in the brain. As a result, researchers can focus their studies, for instance, on the *cognitive* tasks that accompany reading, as distinct from the intricate processing of written words at the purely *visual* level.

With these finer distinctions comes the ability to recognize interacting pathways of information in areas that had been blurred before and to address physiological problems that crop up at specific points along those pathways. Two forms of imaging work particularly well in the brain: PET, with its sensitivity to energy levels, and magnetic resonance imaging (MRI), with its precision of anatomical detail. Other imaging modes offer unique advantages as well: computed tomography, which can clearly distinguish gray and white matter; magnetic resonance spectroscopy, which can measure differing rates of energy metabolism in the course of a disease; magnetic source imaging, which has yielded some of the most precise information to date on the origin of epileptic seizures; and ultrasound imaging, favored for use with newborns.

But the Decade of the Brain is more than a phase of new-and-improved technology; after all, technology is continually being improved. What is novel in the 1990s is the intriguing set of questions that are open to exploration—including some that could not even be framed, much less addressed, as recently as 15 years ago. For example, the role of genetics in several mental disorders was long suspected and is now gaining confirmation, as painstaking studies of heredity covering several generations of afflicted families reveal patterns of inheritance; at the same time, molecular biological studies are closing in on a physical explanation of how particular defects in the genes could ultimately lead to recognizable clinical symptoms. (For a fuller discussion, see Chapters 4 and 5.) The magnificent plasticity of the brain—the great degree to which neuronal connections can be affected by environmental factors—is a topic that has also grown well beyond its origins in the study of the visual system. As will be shown in Chapter 6, plasticity is considered an important principle for understanding the processes that form many other functional areas of the brain as well.

Neuroscience also has its own version of parallel processing, which refers to the brain's ability to take in many kinds of perceptual signals through our five senses and to combine them in meaningful patterns (see Chapter 7). The increasing sophistication of computer technology, together with current work in artificial intelligence, finds application in neuroscientific studies of learning and cognition. And questions about the physical location of memory in the brain, which have puzzled scientists and philosophers since Aristotle, can be posed more precisely, thanks to cell-by-cell studies of how learning takes place in a variety of nervous systems, from some of the very simplest to the highly complex (as discussed in Chapter 8).

A rush of technological innovation has recently converged with the momentum of many years of basic research, so that neuroscience is poised for great advances. Research on the brain has always been respected as a specialized line of inquiry within the life sciences; now it takes its place as a major scientific frontier for our times, bringing together many of the most engaging areas in the study of our own physical nature.

A case in point is a specialized brain cell known as the pyramidal neuron. This neuron predominates in the cerebral cortex, the densely wrinkled sheet of "gray matter" that covers the human brain and regulates many of our sensations, thoughts, and characteristically human abilities. With their large cell bodies and their long axons for transmitting signals, pyramidal neurons are excellently suited to their task of bringing together information from one region of the enormously extensive cortex to another; Dominick Purpura only half-jokingly calls them "the acme of biological cellular evolution on earth." These specialized cells not only *transmit* signals; they also incorporate into their structure a very effective pattern of sites for *receiving* signals. Some of the receptor sites are adapted to take up a specific neurotransmitter that inhibits further activity; other receptor sites (pore-like openings in the cell membrane) may respond specifically to calcium.

Another part of the pyramidal neuron, the dendrites, branches outward from the main body of the cell; each dendrite sports a number of spines for receiving signals. These spines have become a feature of great interest in recent years because of growing evidence that they may take an active part in cellular processes that accompany learning. Moreover, it appears that structural and functional changes occur in the neurons that transmit the signals, as well as in those that receive them. Thus, the cellular mechanisms of learning may entail some restructuring throughout a region. To observe and explain these changes, neuroscientists call on several disciplines: biochemistry, molecular biology, and electrophysiology, to name a few.

THE DEDICATION OF A DECADE

What can "the brain's new science" do for humankind? Fortunately, the answers to this question are many. Purpura offers a few: Neuroscience can tell what the brain is made of—something that everyone alive probably wonders about occasionally—and how it takes shape to begin with; how the brain functions as a healthy system in adulthood, and what happens to it in injury or disease. Following from the last point, further study of the brain can direct researchers and health care professionals toward the prevention of many illnesses, bringing a halt to the ravages that such illnesses visit on millions of patients every year. Enoch Gordis adds another answer: The findings of neuroscience have been vital to recent gains in understanding the addictive disorders, from the genetic and environmental factors that figure into addictions to a clearer view of how drugs (including alcohol) act on the brain and how the injurious cycle of substance abuse can best be treated.

Besides the direct application of its findings, neuroscience offers something that is of the greatest value in advanced research today: an overview. The broad perspective of neuroscience makes it possible to bring together disparate problems under a single unifying principle. Specific problems then fall into place as variations on the common principle, each with its appropriate context and function. An example is the action of lithium on brain cells—well established as an effective treatment for manic-depressive illness, but one whose mode of action is not yet completely understood. The strongest hypothesis at present is that lithium works by interfering with the brain's synthesis of a vitamin called inositol. This substance appears to act as part of a chain of chemical signals that affect mood; as a vitamin, though, it is also crucial in embryonic development, and its blockage during a pregnancy can lead to birth defects. Thus, an older observation—that lithium can be harmful during pregnancy—may be explained by the compound's interference with inositol.

As another example, the level of calcium in cells can vary widely across regions of the brain and is often a major factor in healthy functioning. Many kinds of cells can take up calcium, but some are unable to remove it again (for example, the neurons of the hippocampus, a brain structure thought to be responsible for short-term memory). As a result, calcium accumulates and eventually destroys the cell. The inability to remove calcium may offer a clue to disorders that involve overactivity in certain brain regions, such as epilepsy, and to some degenerative disorders as well. In many other areas of brain research, too, neuroscience provides a unifying principle for tackling a problem from several angles at once: in the study of brain tumors, injuries of the brain and spinal cord, and dementias and other mental disorders that show evidence of some physical as well as psychological basis.

In the opinion of many researchers, another challenge that awaits neuroscience is the examination of human nature itself and of the destructive strain that humankind seems to carry from one generation to the next like an inherited disease. Human history is dense with examples of aggression against our own and other species, for every imaginable reason and in every conceivable form. Perhaps this tendency is an inescapable part of our nature—or, indeed, of any animal nature. When coupled with the endless capabilities of human intelligence, however, it threatens destruction on a scale that would make any further research irrelevant. The challenge is to come to terms with human aggression before it reduces all our possibilities to silence. Neuroscience, with its theoretical, experimental, and clinical perspectives on the human brain and the human mind, can contribute significantly to meeting this challenge.

As mentioned earlier, the Decade of the Brain was launched with a symposium. Under the sponsorship of the Institute of Medicine and the National Institute of Mental Health, many of the world's eminent neuroscientists gathered in July 1990 to discuss some of the exciting results from recent investigations and to plan research strategies for the future—strategies to make the most of the new prospects created by technology and by alliances between the public and private sectors (see Chapter 9). Maxwell Cowan, chief scientific officer of the Howard Hughes Medical Institute and chairman of the symposium's steering committee, listed three objectives for the event.

First, it was a call to celebrate the great achievements in brain research, the years of painstaking work, at times without evident reward, and the advances—some small, some almost revolutionarily large—that have shaped the field during the second half of this century. Second, the symposium was to bring to the attention of policymakers the rich opportunities offered by neuroscience to address so many of the illnesses and disorders that threaten our country's public health, lower our productivity, and bring about great suffering for millions of Americans every year. Vigorous support for further research during the Decade of the Brain will be crucial if neuroscience is to extend today's experimental results into clinical practice and to make possible the results of tomorrow and the next 10 years.

Third, the symposium was an event for the public: a chance for interested people in all fields to learn about the latest work and to share for a day or two in the heady sensation of surveying a scientific frontier together with some of the leading workers who are currently exploring it. The American public has been and continues to be the principal sponsor of scientific research; and in the study of the human brain, in particular, a great share of the field's excitement, as well as a clear presentation of its principles and methods, is owed to the public. This book aims to present both, with a minimum of jargon and with the optimum of interest and accessibility. Not only as sponsors of research, but as living, thinking exemplars of the infinitely varied creativity of the human brain, we are all entitled to share in the promise of neuroscience.

ACKNOWLEDGMENTS

Chapter 1 is based on presentations by Maxwell Cowan, Enoch Gordis, and Dominick Purpura.

2

Major Structures and Functions
of the Brain

Outside the specialized world of neuroanatomy and for most of the uses of daily life, the brain is more or less an abstract entity. We do not experience our brain as an assembly of physical structures (nor would we wish to, perhaps); if we envision it at all, we are likely to see it as a large, rounded walnut, grayish in color.

This schematic image refers mainly to the cerebral cortex, the outermost layer that overlies most of the other brain structures like a fantastically wrinkled tissue wrapped around an orange. The preponderance of the cerebral cortex (which, with its supporting structures, makes up approximately 80 percent of the brain's total volume) is actually a recent development in the course of evolution. The cortex contains the physical structures responsible for most of what we call "brainwork": cognition, mental imagery, the highly sophisticated processing of visual information, and the ability to produce and understand language. But underneath this layer reside many other specialized structures that are essential for movement, consciousness, sexuality, the action of our five senses, and more—all equally valuable to human existence. Indeed, in strictly biological terms, these structures can claim priority over the cere-

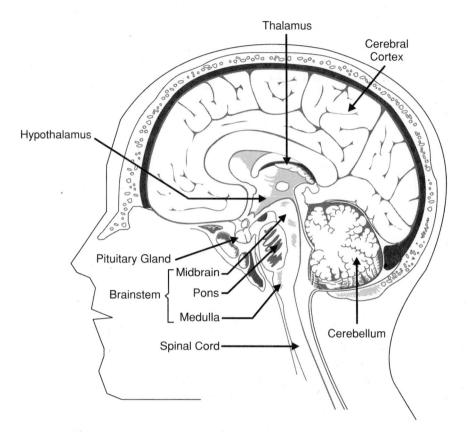

FIGURE 2.1.   The brain owes its outer appearance of a walnut to the wrinkled and deeply folded cerebral cortex, which handles the innumerable signals responsible for perception and movement and also for mental processes.   Below the surface of the cortex are packed a number of other specialized structures: the thalamus, an important relay station for the senses, and the hypothalamus, a meeting point between the nervous system and the endocrine system and between emotion and physical feeling. The pituitary gland, acting on signals from the hypothalamus, produces hormones that regulate many functions from growth to reproduction.   The pons and the medulla, two major elements of the brainstem, channel nerve signals between the brain and other parts of the body, controlling vital functions such as breathing and deliberate movement.   (The extension of this signal pathway throughout the trunk and abdomen is, of course, the spinal cord.)   At the back of the brain is the cerebellum, which coordinates the brain's instructions for skilled repetitive movements and for maintaining posture and balance.   Source: Adapted from G. J. Torbra, *Principles of Human Anatomy,* 3rd ed. Harper and Row (1983).

bral cortex. In the growth of the individual embryo, as well as in evolutionary history, the brain develops roughly from the base of the skull up and outward. The human brain actually has its beginnings, in the four-week-old embryo, as a simple series of bulges at one end of the neural tube.

VENTRICLES

The bulges in the neural tube of the embryo develop into the hindbrain, midbrain, and forebrain—divisions common to all vertebrates, from sharks to squirrels to humans. The original hollow structure is commemorated in the form of the ventricles, which are cavities containing cerebrospinal fluid. During the course of development, the three bulges become four ventricles. In the hindbrain is the fourth ventricle, continuous with the central canal of the spinal cord. A cavity in the forebrain becomes the third ventricle, which leads further forward into the two lateral ventricles, one in each cerebral hemisphere.

BRAINSTEM

The hindbrain contains several structures that regulate autonomic functions, which are essential to survival and not under our conscious control. The brainstem, at the top of the spinal cord, controls breathing, the beating of the heart, and the diameter of blood vessels. This region is also an important junction for the control of deliberate movement. Through the medulla, at the lower end of the brainstem, pass all the nerves running between the spinal cord and the brain; in the pyramids of the medulla, many of these nerve tracts for motor signals cross over from one side of the body to the other. Thus, the left brain controls movement of the right side of the body, and the right brain controls movement of the left side.

In addition to being the major site of crossover for nerve tracts running to and from the brain, the medulla is the seat of several pairs of nerves for organs of the chest and abdomen, for movements of the shoulder and head, for swallowing, salivation, and taste, and for hearing and equilibrium.

At the top of the brainstem is the pons—literally, a bridge—between the lower brainstem and the midbrain. Nerve impulses traversing the pons pass on to the cerebellum (or "little brain"), which is concerned primarily with the coordination of complex muscular movement. In addition, nerve fibers running through the pons relay sensations of touch from the spinal cord to the upper brain centers.

Many nerves for the face and head have their origin in the pons, and these nerves regulate some movements of the eyeball, facial expression, salivation, and taste. Together with nerves of the medulla, nerves from the pons also control breathing and the body's sense of equilibrium.

What had been the middle bulge in the neural tube develops into the midbrain, which functions mainly as a relay center for sensory and motor nerve impulses between the pons and spinal cord and the thalamus and cerebral cortex. Nerves in the midbrain also control some movements of the eyeball, pupil, and lens and reflexes of the eyes, head, and trunk.

THALAMUS AND HYPOTHALAMUS

Deep in the core area of the brain, just above the top of the brainstem, are structures that have a great deal to do with perception, movement, and the body's vital functions. The thalamus consists of two oval masses, each embedded in a cerebral hemisphere, that are joined by a bridge. The masses contain nerve cell bodies that sort information from four of the senses—sight, hearing, taste, and touch—and relay it to the cerebral cortex. (Only the sense of smell sends signals directly to the cortex, bypassing the thalamus.) Sensations of pain, temperature, and pressure are also relayed through the thalamus, as are the nerve impulses from the cerebral hemispheres that initiate voluntary movement.

The hypothalamus, despite its relatively small size (roughly that of a thumbnail), controls a number of drives essential for the functioning of a wide-ranging omnivorous social mammal. At the autonomic level, the hypothalamus stimulates smooth muscle (which lines the blood vessels, stomach, and intestines) and receives sensory impulses from these areas. Thus it controls the rate of the heart, the passage of food through the alimentary canal, and contraction of the bladder.

The hypothalamus is the main point of interaction for the

body's two physical control systems: the nervous system, which transmits information in the form of minute electrical impulses, and the endocrine system, which brings about changes of state through the release of chemical factors. It is the hypothalamus that first detects crucial changes in the body and responds by stimulating various glands and organs to release hormones.

The hypothalamus is also the brain's intermediary for translating emotion into physical response. When strong feelings (rage, fear, pleasure, excitement) are generated in the mind, whether by external stimuli or by the action of thoughts, the cerebral cortex transmits impulses to the hypothalamus; the hypothalamus may then send signals for physiological changes through the autonomic nervous system and through the release of hormones from the pituitary. Physical signs of fear or excitement, such as a racing heartbeat, shallow breathing, and perhaps a clenched "gut feeling," all originate here.

Also in the hypothalamus are neurons that monitor body temperature at the surface through nerve endings in the skin, and other neurons that monitor the blood flowing through this part of the brain itself, as an indicator of core body temperature. The front part of the hypothalamus contains neurons that act to lower body temperature by relaxing smooth muscle in the blood vessels, which causes them to dilate and increases the rate of heat loss from the skin. Through its neurons associated with the sweat glands of the skin, the hypothalamus can also promote heat loss by increasing the rate of perspiration. In opposite conditions, when the body's temperature falls below the (rather narrow) ideal range, a portion of the hypothalamus directs the contraction of blood vessels, slows the rate of heat loss, and causes the onset of shivering (which produces a small amount of heat).

The hypothalamus is the control center for the stimuli that underlie eating and drinking. The sensations that we interpret as hunger arise partly from a degree of emptiness in the stomach and partly from a drop in the level of two substances: glucose circulating in the blood and a hormone that the intestine produces shortly after the intake of food. (Receptors for this hormone gauge how far digestion has proceeded since the last meal.) This system is not a simple "on" switch for hunger, however: another portion of the hypothalamus, when stimulated, actively inhibits eating by promoting a feeling of satiety. In experimental animals, damage to this portion of the brain is associated with continued excessive eating, eventually leading to obesity.

In addition to these numerous functions, there is evidence that the hypothalamus plays a role in the induction of sleep. For one thing, it forms part of the reticular activating system, the physical basis for that hard-to-define state known as consciousness (about which more later); for another, electrical stimulation of a portion of the hypothalamus has been shown to induce sleep in experimental animals, although the mechanism by which this works is not yet known. In all, the hypothalamus is a richly complex cubic centimeter of vital connections, which will continue to reward close study for some time to come. Because of its unique position as a midpost between thought and feeling and between conscious act and autonomic function, a thorough understanding of its workings should tell us much about the earliest history and development of the human animal.

PITUITARY AND PINEAL GLANDS

The pituitary and the pineal glands function in close association with the hypothalamus. The pituitary responds to signals from the hypothalamus by producing an array of hormones, many of which regulate the activities of other glands: thyroid-stimulating hormone, adrenocorticotropic hormone (which stimulates an outpouring of epinephrine in response to stress), prolactin (involved in the production of milk), and the sex hormones follicle-stimulating hormone and luteinizing hormone, which promote the development of eggs and sperm and regulate the timing of ovulation. The pituitary gland also produces several hormones with more general effects: human growth hormone, melanocyte-stimulating hormone (which plays a role in the pigmentation of skin), and dopamine, which inhibits the release of prolactin but is better known as a neurotransmitter (see Chapter 5).

The pineal gland produces melatonin, the hormone associated with skin pigmentation. The secretion of melatonin varies significantly over a 24-hour cycle, from low levels during the day to a peak at night, and the pineal gland has been called a "third eye" because it is controlled by neurons sensitive to light, which originate in the retina of each eye and end in the hypothalamus. In animals with a clear-cut breeding season, the pineal gland is a link between the shifting hours of daylight and the hormonal responses of the hypothalamus, which in turn guide reproductive functions. In humans, who can conceive and give birth throughout the year, the pineal gland plays no known role in reproduction, although there is evidence that melatonin has a share in regulating ovulation.

THE "LITTLE BRAIN" AT THE BACK OF THE HEAD

While autonomic and endocrine functions are being maintained by structures deep inside the brain, another specialized area is sorting and processing the signals required to maintain balance and posture and to carry out coordinated movement. The cerebellum (the term in Latin means "little brain") is actually a derived form of the hindbrain—as suggested by its position at the back of the head, partly tucked under the cerebral hemispheres. In humans, with our almost unlimited repertoire of movement, the cerebellum is accordingly large; in fact, it is the second-largest portion of the brain, exceeded only by the cerebral cortex. Its great surface area is accommodated within the skull by elaborate folding, which gives it an irregular, pleated look. In relative terms, the cerebellum is actually largest in the brain of birds, where it is responsible for the constant streams of information between brain and body that are required for flight.

In humans, the cerebellum relays impulses for movement from the motor area of the cerebral cortex to the spinal cord; from there, they pass to their designated muscle groups. At the same time, the cerebellum receives impulses from the muscles and joints that are being activated and in some sense compares them with the instructions issued from the motor cortex, so that adjustments can be made (this time by way of the thalamus). The cerebellum thus is neither the sole initiator of movement nor a simple link in the chain of nerve impulses, but a site for the rerouting and in some cases refining of instructions for movement. There is evidence, too, that the cerebellum can store a sequence of instructions for frequently performed movements and for skilled repetitive movements—those that we think of as learned "by rote."

The right and left hemispheres of the cerebellum each connect with the nerve tracts from the spinal cord on the *same* side of the body, and with the *opposite* cerebral hemisphere. For example, nerve impulses concerned with movement of the left arm originate in the right cerebral hemisphere, and information about the orientation, speed, and force of the movement is fed back to the right cerebral hemisphere, through the left half of the cerebellum. The nerves responsible for movement at the ends of the arms and legs tend to have their origin near the outer edges of the cerebellum. By contrast, nerves that have their origin near the center of the cerebellum serve to monitor the body's overall orientation in space and to maintain upright posture, in response to information about balance that is transmitted by nerve impulses from the inner ear, among other sources.

RETICULAR NETWORK

Some nerve fibers from the cerebellum also contribute to the reticular formation, a widespread network of neurons ("reticular" is derived from the Latin word for "net"). This formation and some neurons in the thalamus, together with others from various sensory systems of the brain, make up the reticular activating system—the means by which we maintain consciousness. The reticular activating system also comes into play when we deliberately focus our attention, "tuning out" distractions to some degree. At the midline of the brainstem are the raphe nuclei, whose axons extend down into the spinal cord and up to the cerebral cortex—a reach that makes it possible for many areas of the nervous system to be contacted simultaneously. The reticular formation plays a role in movement, particularly those forms of movement that do not call for conscious attention: it is also involved in transmitting or inhibiting sensations of pain, temperature, and touch. Less tangibly, the reticular activating system appears to work as a filter for the countless stimuli that can act on the nervous system both from within and from outside the body. It is this filtering of signals that allows a passenger on an airplane, for example, to doze off undisturbed by sounds of nearby conversation and steady jet engines, but to awake and become alert when the pitch of the engines changes and the plane tilts into its descent.

THE "EMOTIONAL BRAIN"

The limbic system (from the Latin *limbus*, for "hem" or "border") is another assembly of linked structures that form a loose circuit throughout the brain. This system is a fairly old part of the brain and one that humans share with many other vertebrates; in reptiles, it is known as the rhinencephalon, or "smell-brain," because it reacts primarily to signals of odor. In humans, of course, the stimuli that can affect the emotional brain are just about limitless in their variety.

The limbic system is responsible for most of the basic drives and emotions and the associated involuntary behavior that are important for an animal's survival: pain and pleasure, fear, anger, sexual feelings, and even docility and affection. As with the rhinencephalon, the sense of smell is a powerful factor. Nerves from the olfactory bulb, by which all odor is perceived, track directly into the limbic system at several points and are then connected through it to other parts of the brain; hence the ability of pheromones, and perhaps of other odors as well, to influence behavior in quite complex ways without necessarily reaching our conscious awareness.

Also feeding into the limbic system are the thalamus and hypothalamus, as well as the amygdala, a small, almond-shaped complex of nerve cells that receive input from both the olfactory system and the cerebral cortex. These connections are illustrated in an unusual way in the context of epilepsy. Perhaps because the amygdala is located near a common site of origin of epileptic seizures—that is, in the temporal lobe of the cerebral hemispheres—epileptics sometimes experience unidentifiable or unpleasant odors or changes of mood as part of the aura preceding a seizure. The limbic system is not thought to be involved in the causes of epilepsy, but it is indirectly stimulated by the electric discharge in the brain that sets off a seizure and gives evidence of the stimulation in its own characteristic ways.

HIPPOCAMPUS

The hippocampus is another major structure of the limbic system. Named for its fanciful resemblance to the shape of a sea horse, the hippocampus is located at the base of the temporal lobe near several sets of association fibers. These are bundles of nerve fibers that connect one region of the cerebral cortex with another, so that the hippocampus, as well as other parts of the limbic system, exchanges signals with the entire cerebral cortex. The hippocampus has been shown to be important for the consolidation of recently acquired information. (In contrast, long-term memory is thought to be stored throughout the cerebral cortex. The means by which short-term memory is converted into long-term memory has posed a particularly challenging riddle that only now is beginning to yield to investigation; see Chapter 8.)

Recent work with a variety of animals has found dense clusters of receptor sites for tetrahydrocannabinol, the active ingredient of marijuana and related drugs, in the hippocampus and other nearby structures of the limbic system. This localization helps explain the effects of marijuana, which range from mild euphoria to wavering attention to temporarily weakened short-term memory. A loss of short-term memory is also seen in certain syndromes of alcoholism and in Alzheimer's disease, which involves some degeneration of the hippocampus and other limbic structures.

CEREBRAL CORTEX

The cerebral cortex occupies by far the greatest surface area of the human brain and presents its most striking aspect. Also known as the neocortex, this is the most recently evolved area of the brain. In fact, the enormous expansion in the area of the cerebral cortex is hypothesized to have begun only about 2 million years ago, in the earliest members of the genus *Homo*; the result today is a brain weighing approximately three times more than would be expected for a mammal our size. The cortex is named for its resemblance to the bark of a tree, because it covers the surface of the cerebral hemispheres in a similar way. Its wrinkled convoluted appearance is due to a

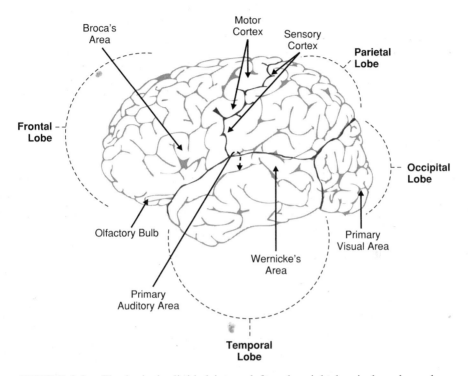

FIGURE 2.2. The brain is divided into a left and a right hemisphere by a deep groove that runs from the front of the head (at left) to the back (at right). In each hemisphere, the cerebral cortex falls into four main divisions, or lobes, set off from one another by noticeable folds in the surface. Although there is some overlap of tasks among the lobes, each is best known for one or two specialized functions. The frontal lobes house the motor area (responsible for instructions of movement) and Broca's area, which handles the production of speech. The faculties of planning and mental representation of the outside world are also attributed to the frontal lobes. In the parietal lobes, the cerebral cortex processes the signals that come from sensation; the temporal lobes are concerned with memory, hearing, and, in Wernicke's area, with the ability to understand language. The occipital lobes are specialized to manage the intricate processing of vision. The olfactory bulb, one of the older parts of the brain in vertebrates, is tucked just under the frontal lobes.

24

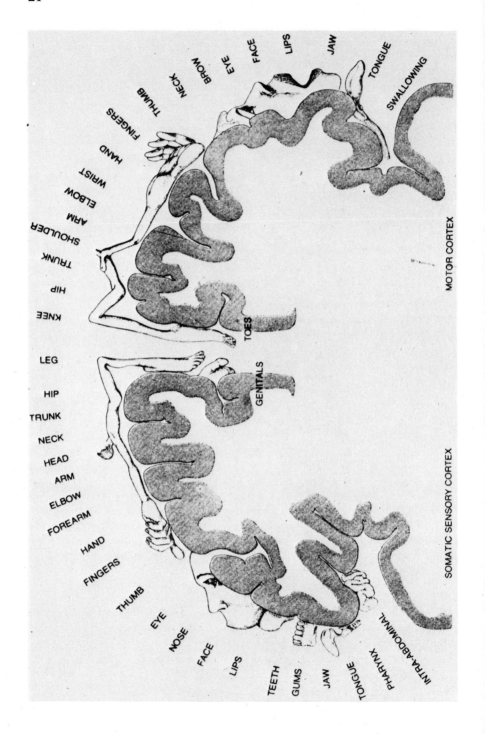

growth spurt during the fourth and fifth months of embryonic development, when the gray matter of the cortex is expanding greatly as its cells grow in size. The supporting white matter, meanwhile, grows less rapidly; as a result, the brain takes on the dense folds and fissures characteristic of an object with great surface area crowded into a small space.

Although the folds in the cerebral cortex appear at first to be random, they include several prominent bulges, or gyri, and grooves, or sulci, that act as landmarks in what is in fact a highly ordered structure (the finer details of which are still not completely known). The deepest groove extends from the front to the back of the head, dividing the brain into the left and right hemispheres. The central sulcus, which runs from the middle of the brain outward to both left and right, and the lateral sulcus, another left-to-right groove somewhat lower on the hemispheres and toward the back of the head, further divide each hemisphere into four lobes: frontal, parietal, temporal, and occipital. A fifth lobe, known as the insula, is located deep within the parietal and temporal lobes and is not apparent as a separate structure on the outer surface of the cerebral hemispheres.

Two noticeable bulges, the precentral gyrus and the postcentral gyrus, are named for their positions just in front of and just behind the central sulcus, respectively. The precentral gyrus is the site of the primary motor area, responsible for conscious movement. From eyebrows to toes, the movable parts of the body are "mapped" on this area of the cortex, with each muscle group or limb represented here by a population of neurons. In complementary fashion, the job of receiving sensations from all parts of the body is managed by the primary somatosensory area, which is located in the postcentral gyrus. Here, too, the human form is mapped, and, as with the precen-

---

FIGURE 2.3. Two miniature "maps" represent the body on the cerebral cortex. One of these, in the motor area, assigns a specific portion of the cortex to each part of the body that calls for muscular control; the portions assigned to the fingers, lips, and tongue are surprisingly large, reflecting the demands of highly precise instructions needed for speech and for manual skills. The other map, in the sensory area, devotes a specific area to each part of the body that receives sensations. Here, again, the portion for the face and hands is relatively large—but so, too, is the portion that processes signals from the abdomen and intestines. Source: W. H. Freeman, 1979. *The Brain: A Scientific American Book.*

tral gyrus, the areas devoted to the hand and the mouth are disproportionately large. Their size reflects the elaborate brain circuitry that makes possible the precision grip of the human hand, the fine motor and sensory signals required for striking up a violin arpeggio or sharpening a tool, and the coordination of the lips, tongue, and vocal apparatus to produce the highly arbitrary and significant sounds of human language.

Close observations of animals and humans after injury to particular sites of the brain indicate that many areas of the cortex control quite specific functions. Additional findings have come from stimulating sites on the cortex with a small electrical charge in experimental procedures or during surgery; the result might be an action in some part of the body (if the motor cortex is involved) or (for a sensory function) a pattern of electrical discharges in other parts of the cortex. Careful exploration has established, for example, that the auditory area in the temporal lobe is made up of smaller regions, each attuned to different sound frequencies.

But for much of the cortex, no such direct functions have been found, and for a time these areas were known as "silent" cortex. It is now clear that "association" cortex is a better name for them because they fill the crucial role of making sense of received stimuli, piecing together the signals from various sensory pathways and making the synthesis available as felt experience. For instance, if there is to be not merely perception but conscious understanding of sounds, the auditory association area (just behind the auditory area proper) must be active. In the hemisphere that houses speech and other verbal abilities—the left hemisphere, for most people—the auditory association area blends into the receptive language area (which also receives signals from the visual association area, thereby providing a neural basis for reading as well as for the comprehension of speech in most languages).

A large portion of the association cortex is found in the frontal lobes, which have expanded most rapidly over the past 20,000 or so generations (about 500,000 years) of human evolution. Medical imaging shows increased activity in the association cortex after other areas of the brain have received electrical stimulation and also before the initiation of movement. On present evidence, it is in the association cortex that we locate long-term planning, interpretation, and the organization of ideas—perhaps the most recently developed elements of the modern human brain.

Visual functions occupy the occipital lobe, the bulge at the back end of the brain. The primary area for visual perception is almost surrounded by the much larger visual association area. Nearby, extending into the lower part of the temporal lobe, is the association area for visual *memory*—a specialized area in the cortex. Clearly, this function has been important for an omnivorous foraging primate that probably spent a long evolutionary period ranging among scattered food sources. (For an account of the intricate mechanisms that underlie depth perception and color vision, see Chapter 7.)

A less specific kind of function has been attributed to the prefrontal cortex, located on the forward-facing part of the frontal lobes. This area is connected by association fibers with all other regions of the cortex and also with the amygdala and the thalamus, which means that it, too, makes up part of the "emotional brain," the limbic system. Injury to the prefrontal cortex or its underlying white matter results in a curious disability: the patient suffers from a reduced intensity of emotion and can no longer foretell the consequences of things that are said or done. (The injury must be bilateral to produce such an effect; if only one hemisphere is injured, the other can compensate and avert this strange, potentially crippling social deficit.) Among its other functions, the prefrontal cortex is responsible for inhibiting inappropriate behavior, for keeping the mind focused on goals, and for providing continuity in the thought process.

Long-term memory has not yet been found to reside in any exclusive part of the brain, but experimental findings indicate that the temporal lobes contribute to this function. Electrical stimulation of the cerebral cortex in this area gives rise to sensations of déjà vu ("already seen") and its opposite, jamais vu ("never seen"); it also conjures up images of scenes witnessed or speech heard in the past. That the association areas for vision and hearing and the language areas are all nearby may suggest pathways for the storage and retrieval of memories that include several types of stimuli.

The function of language itself is housed in the left hemisphere (in most cases), in several discrete sites on the cortex.

The expressive language area, responsible for the production of speech, is found toward the center of the frontal lobe; this is also called Broca's area, after the French anatomist and anthropologist of the mid-1800s who was among the first to observe differences in function between the left and right hemispheres. The receptive language area, which is located near the junction of the parietal and temporal lobes, allows us to comprehend both spoken and written language, as described above. This is often called Wernicke's area, after the German neurologist Karl Wernicke, who in the late 1800s laid the basis for much of our current understanding of how the brain encodes and decodes language. A bundle of nerve fibers connects Wernicke's area directly to Broca's area. This tight linkage is important, since before any speech at all can be uttered, its form and appropriate words must first be assembled in Wernicke's area and then relayed to Broca's area to be mentally translated into the requisite sounds; only then can it pass to the supplementary motor cortex for vocal production.

For nine of ten right-handed people and almost two-thirds of all left-handers, language abilities are sited in the left hemisphere. No one knows why there should be this asymmetrical distribution rather than an even balance or, for that matter, a consistent location of language in the left brain. What is clear is that in all cases, the hemisphere that does *not* contain language abilities holds the key to other functions of a less distinct, more holistic nature. The appreciation of forms and textures, the recognition of the timbre of a voice, and the ability to orient oneself in space all appear to lodge here, as do musical talent and appreciation—a host of perceptions that do not lend themselves well to analysis in words.

The limited specialization of the two hemispheres is efficient in terms of the use of space: it increases the functional abilities of the brain without adding to its volume. (The skull of the human infant, it is calculated, is already as large as can be accommodated through the birth canal, which in turn is constrained by the skeletal requirements for upright walking.) Moreover, the bilateral arrangement allows for some flexibility if one hemisphere is injured; often the other hemisphere can compensate to some degree, depending on the age at which injury occurs (a young, still-developing brain readjusts more readily).

The two hemispheres are connected mainly by a thick bundle of nerve fibers called the corpus callosum, or "hard body," because of its tough consistency. A smaller bundle, the anterior commissure, connects just the two temporal lobes. Although the corpus callosum is a good landmark for students of brain anatomy, its contribution to behavior has been difficult to pin down. Patients in whom the corpus callosum has been severed (a way of ameliorating epilepsy by restricting seizures to one side of the brain) go about their everyday business without impairment. Careful testing does turn up a gap between sensations processed by the right brain and the language centers of the left brain—for instance, a person with a severed corpus callosum is unable to name an object placed unseen in the left hand (because stimuli perceived by the left half of the body are processed in the right hemisphere). On the whole, though, it appears that the massive crossing-over of nerve fibers that takes place in the brainstem is quite adequate for most purposes, at least those related to survival.

Although the cerebral cortex is quite thin, ranging from 1.5 to 4 millimeters deep (less than 3/8 inch), it contains no fewer than six layers. From the outer surface inward, these are the molecular layer, made up for the most part of junctures between neurons for the exchange of signals; the external granular layer, mainly interneurons, which serve as communicating nerve bodies within a region; an external pyramidal layer, with large-bodied "principal" cells whose axons extend into other regions; an internal granular layer, the main termination point for fibers from the thalamus; a second, internal pyramidal layer, whose cells project their axons mostly to structures below the cortex; and a multiform layer, again containing principal cells, which in this case project to the thalamus. The layers vary in thickness at different sites on the cortex; for example, the granular layers (layers 2 and 4) are more prominent in the primary sensory area and less so in the primary motor area.

BUILDING BLOCKS OF THE BRAIN

Extensive and intricate as the human brain is, and with the almost limitless variation of which it is capable, it is built from relatively few basic units. The fundamental building block of the human brain, like that of nervous systems throughout the animal kingdom, is the neuron, or nerve cell. The neuron conducts signals by means of an axon, which extends outward from the soma, or body of the cell, like a single long arm. Numerous shorter arms, the dendrites ("little branches"), conduct signals back to the soma.

The ability of the axon to conduct nerve impulses is greatly enhanced by the myelin sheath that surrounds it, interrupted at intervals by nodes. Myelin is a fatty substance, a natural electrical insulator, that protects the axon from interference by other nearby nerve impulses. The arrangement of nodes increases the speed of conductivity, so that an electrical impulse sent along the axon can literally jump from node to node, reaching velocities as high as 120 meters per second.

The site of communication between any two neurons—actually not a physical contact but an infinitesimal cleft across which signals are transmitted—is called a synapse, from the Greek word for "conjunction." An axon may extend over a variable distance to make contact with other neurons at a synapse. The end of an axon near a synapse widens out into a bouton, or button; the bouton contains mitochondria, which supply energy, and a number of synaptic vesicles. It is these vesicles, each less than 200 billionths of a meter in diameter, that contain the chemical neurotransmitters to be released into the synaptic cleft. On the other side of the synapse is usually a dendrite, sometimes with a dendritic spine—a small protuberance that expands the surface area of the dendrite and provides a receptive site for incoming signals.

A completely different arangement for transmitting signals is the electrical synapse, at which the cell membranes of two neurons are extremely close together and are linked by a bridge of tubular protein molecules. This bridge allows passage of water and electrically charged small molecules; any change in electrical charge in one neuron is instantaneously transmitted to the other. Hence this mechanism for relaying signals relies entirely on direct electrical coupling; an electrical synapse is about 3 nanometers (nm), or billionths of a meter, wide, as compared with the 25-nm gap of a chemical synapse. Outside of nervous tissue, electrical synapses (and other, similar gap junctions) are the messengers of choice.

The brain is sometimes said to be full of "gray matter," which is supposed to be the stuff of intelligence. The material referred to is actually grayish pink in living brain, and only gray in specimens that have been chemically preserved; it consists of nerve cell bodies and dendrites and the origins and boutons of axons. It is gray matter that forms sheets of cortex on the surface of the cerebral hemispheres. White matter receives its name from the appearance of the myelin enclosing the elongated region of axons. The third main form of matter in the brain is the neuroglia, or "glue" cells. These cells do not connect the neurons, as their name implies; connections are already far from scarce, with the vast system of neural soma, axons, and dendrites packed so densely into the brain. Rather, the neuroglia provide structural support and a source of metabolic energy for the roughly 100 billion nerve cells of the human brain.

CHEMICAL AND ELECTRICAL SIGNALS

The actual signals transmitted throughout the brain come in two forms, electrical and chemical. The two forms are interdependent and meet at the synapse, where chemical substances can alter the electrical conditions within and outside the cell membrane.

A nerve cell at rest holds a slight negative charge (about –70 millivolts, or thousandths of a volt, mV) with respect to the exterior; the cell membrane is said to be polarized. The negative charge, the resting potential of the membrane, arises from a very slight excess of negatively charged molecules inside the cell.

A membrane at rest is more or less impermeable to positively charged sodium ions (Na^+), but when stimulated it is transiently open to their passage. The Na^+ ions thus flow in, attracted by the negative charge inside, and the membrane temporarily reverses its polarity, with a higher positive charge inside than out. This stage lasts less than a millisecond, and then the sodium channels close again. Potassium channels (K^+) open, and K^+ ions move out through the membrane, reversing the flow of positively charged ions. (Both these channels are known as voltage-gated, meaning that they open or close in response to changes in electrical charge occurring across the membrane.) Over the next 3 milliseconds, the membrane becomes slightly hyperpolarized, with a charge of about –80 mV, and then returns to its resting potential. During this time the sodium channels remain closed; the membrane is in a refractory phase.

An action potential—the very brief pulse of positive membrane voltage—is transmitted forward along the axon; it is prevented from propagating backward as long as the sodium channels remain closed. After the membrane has returned to its resting potential, however, a new impulse may arrive to evoke an action potential, and the cycle can begin again.

Gated channels, and the concomitant movement of ions in and out of the cell membrane, are widespread throughout the nervous system, with sodium, potassium, and chlorine being the most common ions involved. Calcium channels are also important, particularly at the presynaptic boutons of axons. When the membrane is at its resting potential, positively charged calcium ions (Ca^{2+}) outside the cell far outnumber those inside. With the advent of an action potential, however, calcium ions rush into the cell. The influx of calcium ions leads to the release of neurotransmitter into the synaptic cleft; this passes the signal to a neighboring nerve cell.

Having taken a close look at the electrical side of the picture, we are in a better position to see where the chemistry comes in. Molecules of neurotransmitter are released into a synaptic cleft and bind to specific receptor sites on the postsynaptic side (the dendrite or dendritic spine), thereby *altering the ion channels* in the postsynaptic membrane. Some neurotransmitters cause sodium channels to open, allowing the influx of Na^+ ions and thus a lessening of negative charge inside the cell membrane. If a considerable number of these potentials are received within a short interval, they can depolarize the membrane enough to trigger an action potential; the result is the transmission of a nerve impulse. The substances that can cause this to occur are the excitatory neurotransmitters. By contrast, other chemical compounds cause potassium channels to open, increasing the outflow of K^+ ions from the cell and making excitation less likely; the neurotransmitters that bring about this state are considered inhibitory.

A given neuron has a great quantity of sites available on its dendrites and cell body and receives signals from many synapses simultaneously, both excitatory and inhibitory. These signals often amount to a rough balance; it is only when the net potential of the membrane in one region shifts significantly up or down from the resting level that a particular neurotransmitter can be said to be exerting an effect. Interestingly, in the membrane's overall balance sheet, the importance of a particular synapse varies with its proximity to where the axon leaves the nerve cell body, so that numerous excitatory potentials out at the ends of the dendrites may be overruled by several inhibitory potentials closer to the soma. Other kinds of synapse regulate the release of neurotransmitters into the synaptic cleft, where they go on to affect the postsynaptic channels as described above.

The list of known neurotransmitters, once thought to be quite short, continues to grow as more substances are found to be synthesized by neurons, contained in presynaptic boutons, and bound on the postsynaptic membrane by specific receptors. Despite stringent requirements for identifying a substance as a neurotransmitter (see Chapter 5), well over two dozen have been so named, and another several dozen strong candidates are under review.

The most cursory look at the human brain can excite awe at its complex functions, the intricacy of its structure, and the innumerable connections all maintained on microscopic fibers a few millionths of a meter in diameter. But a slightly more intimate acquaintance with this 3-pound organ inside our heads, an acquaintance that builds on observation of the brain in action and discovery of the principles by which it works, can yield something more satisfying than awe: the sense of mastery and of rewarded curiosity that comes with understanding. With the rewarding of curiosity as our goal, let us take a closer look at a few aspects of the functioning brain.

3

Glimpses of the Living Brain

Encased in a bony vault and wrapped in layers of tough membrane, the brain has long been considered the most inaccessible of human organs. For centuries, this spongy mass that controls an astonishing array of functions was off limits to medical examination except in the most dire circumstances: grievous injury, surgery undertaken as a last, desperate measure, or postmortem dissection. In all these instances, of course, the brain was very far from its usual level of functioning, and so it was never clear how much these studies could contribute to an understanding of the "normal" brain. Surgeries, autopsies, and neurological examinations of people who had survived brain injury or stroke offered rich details, but the full view of an awake, behaving human brain has continued to tantalize and elude researchers until very recently. In only the past 20 years, options for medical imaging of the brain have increased tremendously, using everything from magnetic waves to charged subatomic particles to computer algorithms as a means of allowing clinicians and researchers to "see" the living brain at work.

THE BRIGHT IMAGES OF PET

Of the many imaging techniques in use today, each has its limits and its strengths. Such factors as cost, labor intensiveness, and fineness of detail in the image help to determine the best uses for each form of imaging, whether in research or in clinical practice. One technique that shows promise in both areas, but that has made a name for itself thus far primarily in research, is positron emission tomography, or PET.

A PET scan measures the distribution in the body of a radioactively "labeled" substance that the patient has received shortly before the scan. Adding a radioactive label to compounds such as glucose (the main source of energy for the brain) permits researchers to the monitor metabolism—roughly, the rate at which energy is being used, or the rate of activity going on—at particular sites. Brain cells take up the radioactively tagged glucose for use; the glucose is metabolized, and the transiently radioactive atoms remain inside the cells, giving off positively charged particles. These "positrons" quickly collide with nearby electrons, then give rise to gamma radiation, which can be detected outside the body and mapped by a computer.

The resulting image of the brain, which is often enhanced with color to make the different values easier to see, quite clearly distinguishes those parts of the brain that are using more glucose from those that are using less. Thus PET can show where nerve cells are more active and where they are less so, not only in cases of disease or disorder but during a particular task or thought or emotion. As an even more flexible measurement of function in the normal brain, PET can detect changes in local blood flow. Small blood vessels respond very rapidly to the needs of nerve cells, axons, and dendrites, so that a full scan's worth of information can be gathered in 40 seconds, as compared with the 45 minutes required to measure glucose metabolism.

Although the PET scan may be familar to most readers as a series of still pictures, the technique is in fact highly dynamic and well suited to giving an ongoing picture of moment-by-moment changes in the working brain. In this aspect it borrows from several earlier techniques that were developed to show ongoing processes in the body—for example, autoradiography, which used a radioactive tracer to make visible the circulation of blood or the metabolism of energy sources in the brain.

Researchers must also have some independent means of siting the information from a PET scan, perhaps with a few landmarks for comparison, if the moving, changeable images traced by the computer are to have any accuracy with reference to a living three-dimensional brain. Therefore, before a PET scan, the patient or the research subject may be fitted with a mask and given an x-ray. The skull x-ray is useful in two ways: it reveals the overall anatomy of the individual's brain, which will allow for more precise orienting of the PET images, and it can be entered in a computer and "molded" to fit a standardized version of the brain, so that the information from a particular scan can be applied toward a more general understanding of brain anatomy. The resolution of the x-ray is good enough—down to a few millimeters—that researchers can confidently identify a small focus of activity within a subarea (such as the primary visual cortex).

Pinpointing the site of activity is not the only challenge posed by a PET scan. There is also the need to distinguish between slight but meaningful shifts in activity and random irregularities, or background "noise." To take the primary visual cortex as an example, a bright light flashed in the subject's eyes evokes an unmistakable peak of activity visible in a PET image; but a less drastic stimulus, such as a word or two appearing on a screen, will act on nerve cells in the brain much less vigorously, and the corresponding PET image will be harder to read. Moreover, the response may be dispersed among several areas, perhaps those having to do with learning and memory, language, and emotion, as well as the areas containing the visual receptors that must take in the stimulus to begin with. To find subtle responses that might otherwise be overlooked, PET researchers borrow the statistical technique of aggregating the data from a small group of subjects and averaging the responses over the group as a whole. Many of the random signals thus cancel out one another, and the responses that are meaningful show up more clearly.

Armed with the technology to observe local patterns of activity in the brain as they are taking place and a statistical approach for uncovering some of the more subtle signals, PET researchers began in the 1980s to look for research questions worthy of their new technological capabilities. The laboratory of Marcus Raichle, at Washington University School of Medicine, is one that chose to examine how the brain handles language—a fundamentally human feature.

As with any inviting area of research, the first task was to define specifically what would be studied. From the new perspective of the PET scanner, many appealing interrelated aspects of human language abilities called for investigation. If any progress were to be made in unraveling the larger riddles, it could only come from focusing on a series of smaller questions, one or two at a time. So, rather than having subjects perform a complex, multilevel task such as reciting the days of the week—which would call for the active participation of at least half a dozen separate brain areas, even if carried out "unthinkingly"—Raichle and his colleagues decided to start at the other end of the scale. They would begin with as simple a stimulus as possible and build up to more complex stimuli. In fact, the first step was to offer a stimulus that had nothing to do with language but was simply a shape on a screen. This would provide a baseline, showing what the PET scan would look like when the subject was merely sitting at rest under experimental conditions, watching. The levels of activity measured by PET at this stage could be subtracted from all later stages as having nothing to do with the processing of language.

The next stage was the simplest possible presentation of language: asking the subject just to look while words appeared on a screen. The visual cortex is active for this task, as are several other regions, and the pattern of activity that appears is much more extensive than that elicited by showing a plain nonverbal shape. The newly active regions are indeed known to handle language; yet, they clearly cannot comprise *all* of the language areas, for when words are presented for the subject to hear, rather than to view, the parts of the brain that respond are completely different. Still other areas become active if the task is expanded so that the subject does not merely see or hear the word but must produce its meaning.

Raichle's group took a "building-block" approach to this

riddle, choosing to separate out the purely visual aspects of the brain's response to the appearance of a word on a screen. The researchers presented subjects first with arbitrary symbols having the characteristic shapes and angles of letters; next with real letters grouped into units about the length of average words but unpronounceable; then, with strings of letters that looked like normal words and that could be pronounced but happened not to be words in the English language; and finally, with authentic English words. A typical sequence might look like this:

$$\nabla \, \varDelta \; \Phi \; \Gamma \; \lrcorner$$
$$\text{N L P F Z}$$
$$\text{T W E A L}$$
$$\text{B O A R D}$$

The goal was to single out very specifically, according to the subjects' responses rather than any preconceived schema, the elements of the brain that responded to written language (as opposed to those that analyze visual patterns, for example). The findings were dramatic: an area known as the medial extrastriate cortex on the left side of the brain came smartly into action as the tasks reached the third and fourth levels (those of pronounceable nonwords and of real words). This was consistent with findings, from a number of earlier studies, that brain injuries at this site interfered with the ability to read words, although they often did not affect speaking or even writing.

Such a pattern of activity, however robust, presumably must be learned rather than innate. One would hardly suppose that the brain is genetically programmed to respond to the sight of graphic symbols that look like words, in English or in any other language. What this means for the researcher is that it may be possible, in long-term studies, to observe the first stirrings of such a response in infants, small children, those just learning the rules of reading, and so on. Ultimately, the goal is to explain just how the ability to comprehend visual word form develops in this exceedingly plastic, versatile territory of the human brain. The benefits to be derived from understanding this process could be very great for the millions of Americans who struggle with dyslexia and other learning disorders.

In addition to exploring the visual aspects of reading, Raichle's

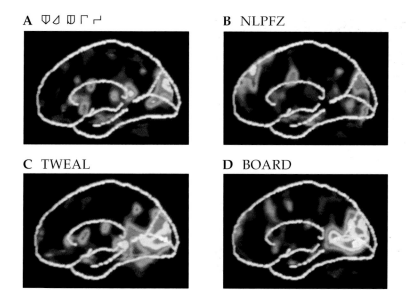

A ▽◁ ◫ Γ ⌐   B NLPFZ

C TWEAL   D BOARD

PLATE 1. As a research subject is shown a series of images on a screen that run from letter-like graphics (A) to a meaningless string of letters (B) to something that is pronounceable but is not a word in English (C) to a real English word (D), several sites come into action or drop out of participation. A positron emission tomographic (PET) image shows activity in the occipital lobe that increases sharply when the graphics become real words. Source: Marcus Raichle, Washington University School of Medicine, St. Louis, Mo.

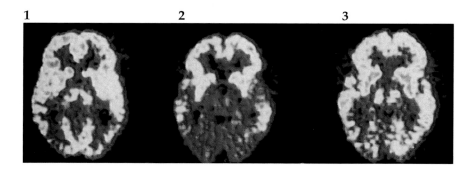

1   2   3

PLATE 2. Treatment with AZT can help in the management of AIDS-related dementia, as is demonstrated by these three PET images. In the healthy brain (1), levels of activity are relatively even through the frontal, temporal, and occipital lobes. Brain activity of a patient with AIDS-related dementia (2) is uneven, with the occipital region and part of the temporal lobes much less active. After 13 weeks of treatment with AZT (3), brain activity has returned significantly toward the normal pattern. Source: National Cancer Institute, Bethesda, Md.

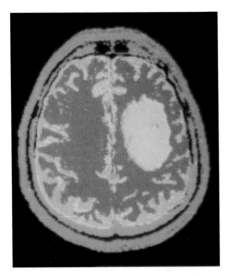

PLATE 3. Magnetic resonance imaging (MRI) is an invaluable tool in clinical practice today, as well as in neuroscientific research. Here, the cross-sectional image of a patient's head clearly discloses the shape and location of a tumor (the egg-shaped yellow mass in the right hemisphere). Healthy brain tissue appears in gray, and the skull and scalp in pink. Such images contribute to precise diagnosis and, when necessary, the planning of neurosurgery.

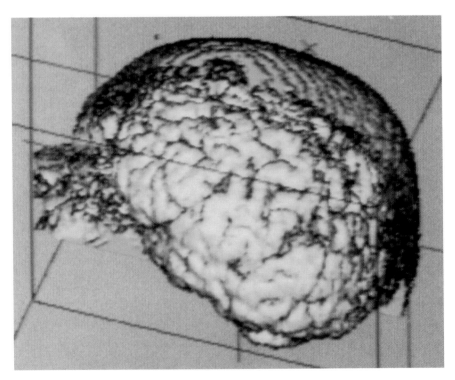

PLATE 4. In further MRI of the patient shown in Plate 3, the surface of the brain is revealed by selectively "cutting away" the scalp.

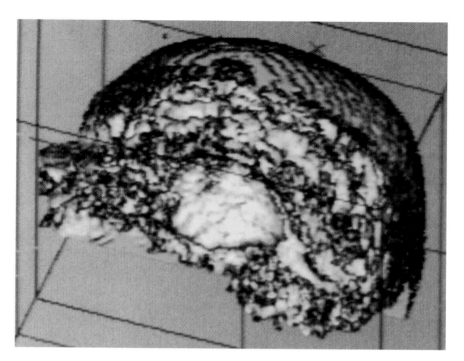

PLATE 5. The brain itself is then cut away, in imaging terms, slice by slice, until the image plane arrives at the tumor. Source for Plates 3–5: H. E. Cline et al., 1990. *Journal of Computer Assisted Tomography* 14(6):1037–1045.

PLATE 6. The positron emission tomographic (PET) scan of a research subject undergoing a panic attack shows very high activity (white area) in a portion of the limbic system, the "emotional brain." What this image of just one hemisphere cannot show, however, is another striking feature of the brains of people subject to panic attacks: an asymmetry between the two hemi-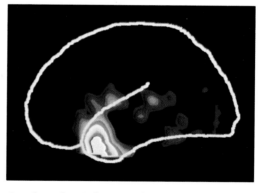spheres, with the left side less active than the right. PET has been useful as a research tool in revealing general patterns of brain activity that characterize panic disorder. Source: Marcus Raichle, Washington University School of Medicine, St. Louis, Mo.

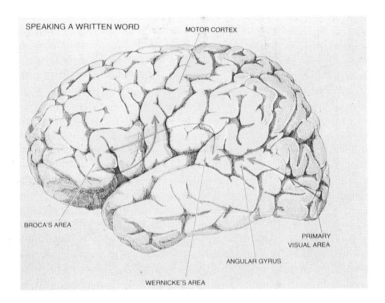

SPEAKING A WRITTEN WORD   MOTOR CORTEX

BROCA'S AREA

PRIMARY
VISUAL AREA

ANGULAR GYRUS

WERNICKE'S AREA

PLATE 7. The simple act of pronouncing a written word is the outcome of an intricate path of signals through several parts of the brain. Recognizing the word calls for the participation of the primary visual area and the visual association areas (in and around the angular gyrus). Then, for the production of speech, Broca's area becomes active; finally, the signals arrive at the motor cortex, which sends instructions for movement to the lips and tongue and larynx. Source: Marcus Raichle, Washington University School of Medicine, St. Louis, Mo.

PLATE 8. At several years of age, humans perform the unusual feat of developing an entirely new visual pathway in their brain: the ability to process written information. The pathway, reinforced by training, can become very strong, even overriding other forms of visual information. To test the dominance of this pathway, try saying aloud the colors in the list. Which word presents itself: the color in which the word appears, or the color name that is written? This test demonstrates the Stroop effect, a well-known psychological phenomenon (see page 120 for additional discussion). Source: Marcus Raichle, Washington University School of Medicine, St. Louis, Mo.

Color names
green
yellow
black
red
green
yellow
blue
black
red
blue

group also designed a building-block series of tasks dealing with the sounds of words (see Plate 1). First, subjects were simply shown pairs of words; then they were shown pairs of words and asked to judge whether they rhymed. The subjects also had to read aloud words that appeared on the screen at the quick pace of one per second.

As the tasks gained in complexity, additional areas of the brain became active. And still further areas became active for tasks that required subjects to turn their attention to the meaning of the words: not only a few sites in the left frontal lobe, in or near the so-called association areas that process many modes of information, but also—and this was a surprise—several sites in the cerebellum. This finding was unexpected because the cerebellum is best known for many functions that are far removed from language: the coordination of movement, fine manual skills, repetitive physical tasks, and so on.

Strikingly, the areas that are active do not remain at their original high levels but actually change and rearrange themselves as the subject becomes more familiar with the task. In terms of behavior, in the course of learning a particular task, there is clearly a point at which the subject begins to make fewer errors and perform the task more fluently. PET scans reveal that internally, too, the brain's functions follow a dynamic course, marking what appears to be the same threshold of familiarity. The left frontal sites and the cerebellum drop out of action as the task is mastered.

These observations begin to suggest new ideas about how the brain at first tackles and then masters a new task—with implications, perhaps, for methods of teaching in a wide variety of subjects that call for well-learned performance.

MEDICAL IMAGES OF EMOTION

Positron emission tomography is not limited to images of learning and motor function. Because it permits close observation of how the brain is using energy, for whatever function, PET actually allows researchers to map what may be called the anatomy of an emotion, in terms of activity patterns in the brain. A topic well suited to this approach is the study of panic disorder, because the behavioral and physiological aspects of the disorder have been well characterized and provide consistent criteria for study. In addition, with the consent of intrepid volunteers who suffer from this disorder, a panic attack can actually be brought on at will in the laboratory, under controlled conditions, by an infusion of sodium lactate. The advantages of laboratory observation are several: the scanning equipment can be set up in advance and timed so as to obtain the maximum information from the panicking subjects in the shortest possible time; and many extraneous factors that might otherwise appear to be associated with a panic attack can, in this neutral setting, be ruled out.

For the Washington University group, eager to see what PET could reveal about panic disorder, the first question was: How does "normal" anxiety (that which would be felt by most individuals, to varying degrees, in a stressful situation) compare with the overwhelming anxiety that is experienced for no discernible reason in a panic attack? The researchers elicited "normal" anxiety in subjects not affected by panic disorder by telling them that they were about to receive an electric shock. (In fact, the measurements were first taken and then a small electric charge was delivered afterward, simply to keep the procedure credible for the subject—otherwise there would be no anxiety and nothing to measure.) The PET scans of normal subjects who went along with this procedure showed patterns of activity in the brain that were much like those of an attack of panic disorder. It is as if the brain produces the state felt as "panic" by one main route regardless of the cause, be it external or internal.

Why then do feelings and physical symptoms of panic mount to the level of a near-crippling disorder in some individuals? PET scans offer some clues about the physical basis of a predisposition toward panic attacks. In a resting, nonpanic state, the brains of panic-disorder sufferers consistently show an asymmetry of blood flow and oxygen use in the two halves of the brain, with the left hemisphere measuring lower on both counts. The site of this asymmetry is known as the parahippocampal gyrus; with its close connections to the hippocampus, it figures largely in the processing of emotional states (see the discussion of the limbic system, the "emotional brain," in Chapter 2).

The particular form of the asymmetry, too, which gives the effect of increased metabolism in the right hemisphere over the left, is intriguing in itself, because a number of other studies have suggested that the right hemisphere is strongly responsible for mental arousal, attention, anxiety, and physiological readiness to respond. Further studies using PET imaging and behavioral measures as well as other approaches should improve our understanding of the physical basis for anxiety, and also of specialization in the two hemispheres of the brain and the physiological circuits underlying emotion.

Other mental disorders are also open to investigation with PET, but they may call for a different experimental approach, because they offer no known "control state." In other words, there may not be a way to reliably induce the characteristic emotion in the laboratory, as sodium lactate can reliably bring on a panic attack in a subject who suffers from panic disorder. Raichle and his co-workers have begun to look at depression with PET; they obtained PET scans from a number of people who had been diagnosed with chronic depression and from a psychiatrically screened, nondepressed population. In comparing the two groups, the researchers found that depressed subjects exhibited less activity than normal subjects in a deep region of the brain known as the caudate nucleus; in a small area of the left frontal cortex and in the limbic system in general, however, activity was increased. The findings were quite specific and corresponded well with other evidence that has turned up in the past few years about physiological factors in depression.

More of a surprise, however, and suggestive of new avenues of investigation was the next experiment. The researchers brought "normal" nondepressed subjects into the laboratory and asked them to think about something sad. This time the resulting PET scans resembled those of the depressed patients: they showed the same site of increased activity in the left frontal cortex. If the same local pattern of reduced activity in the brain holds true both for long-term clinical depression and for transient feelings of sadness, this observation may point toward new ways of exploring both the disabling ailment of depression and the physiological basis for healthy feelings of sadness.

THE X-RAY TODAY

Not only PET but virtually every form of medical imaging can be understood as an attempt to relate an object in space (whose size might range from the entire brain down to a single cell) to events occurring in time (from the human life span down to fractions of a second). The workhorses of medical imaging for most of this century have done a good job on one or the other of these dimensions, addressing either space or time with great precision. X-ray technology, for example, produces highly readable images with fine resolution of detail down to 0.1 millimeter, but these images are static and show only existing structures rather than ongoing processes. On the other hand, electroencephalography, or EEG, which detects small shifts in electric potential at the surface of the skull, measures overall activity of the brain in real time but indicates only roughly *where* in the brain the information is coming from. (Nevertheless, EEG has produced "images," in the form of characteristic patterns of waves, that are useful for study of an aroused or relaxed mental state, of certain phases of sleep, and of a few disorders such as epilepsy and brain tumors.)

The structure of the brain is so intricate, with its folds and fissures, overlapping connections, and underlying compartments, that a clear view of the spatial organization of these 1,400 or so cubic centimeters is crucial for understanding the many ways that disease can affect the brain. For a long time, conventional x-rays fell short on this criterion, because to produce an image on a sheet of film, they necessarily reduced a three-dimensional structure to two dimensions. But the newer version of x-ray imaging gets around this problem with the help of a computer.

Computed tomography uses many x-ray transmissions, sometimes more than a thousand, to produce an image. Each transmission passes an x-ray through the brain at a slightly different angle; integrating all this information is the job of the computer. Because each exposure gives a "tomogram," a rotating view centered on a single axis through an anatomical structure, the three-dimensionality of the body can be pieced together by summing up the different views. Thus, clear, sharp images can be built up by the computer from many tomograms, with unmistakable distinctions among the brain's gray matter or cortex, its white matter (made up largely of myelin sheaths enclosing the nerve branches), and its fluid-filled ventricles.

The practical limitations of computed tomography are built into the technology itself, and it appears unlikely that they will be overcome in the near future. For one thing, the resolution of detail in areas smaller than about 0.5 millimeter is precluded by the focal spot of the x-ray tube, which can never be reduced entirely to a point, and by the x-ray dose itself, which must be kept to a healthy minimum. Another limitation is that x-ray tomograms can show only the comparative densities of various structures; thus they may be very helpful in disease states that affect the overall size or shape of body tissues, but they offer little information on maladies that leave the boundaries of a particular structure unchanged. Within these limits, computed tomography will continue to be used widely for imaging the brain, particularly for possible diagnoses of brain hemorrhage, stroke, or disorders involving the cerebral ventricles.

CREATING PICTURES FROM MAGNETIC WAVES AND SOUND WAVES

A trio of imaging techniques are based on the highly specific ways in which different cells of the body respond to magnetic waves. The best known of the three techniques is magnetic resonance imaging (MRI), in which the patient is actually positioned inside a large magnet (see Plates 3–5). The magnetic field acting on the patient is just powerful enough to bring the magnetic poles of the hydrogen nuclei in the body into alignment. When a single strong pulse of radio waves is fired, the nuclei are knocked into disarray but then realign under the influence of the magnetic field. As they do so, the various types of cells emit a distinct radio signal of their own, which a computer transduces into a visual image.

Different kinds of tissue are distinguished by MRI not on the basis of their density, as with x-ray imaging, but according to the levels of hydrogen they contain. Since hydrogen is found most often as a component of water in the body, the image is largely of structures with different water contents. Tissues with little water content appear bright. Thus fatty tissues show up as bright areas, whereas fluid-filled spaces appear quite dark. MRI produces highly readable images in any plane desired, which is especially helpful for an irregularly shaped mass such as the brain. The contrast among various tissues is often stronger than with x-ray images, although the resolution of detail is not as fine, perhaps about 2 millimeters on the average. Because gray matter has many fluid-containing cell bodies, whereas white matter has more fatty tissue, MRI shows a clear distinction between gray and white matter. The technique is particularly suitable for diagnosing and monitoring the course of such a disease as multiple sclerosis, which affects the fatty myelin sheath enclosing the nerves. MRI is also good for defining the precise location and extent of tumors.

Similar to MRI, and using much of the same equipment and procedures, is magnetic resonance spectroscopy (MRS). Here the magnet and radio waves are "tuned" for atoms other than hydrogen. Phosphorous atoms, for example, form part of phosphate molecules, which are involved in energy metabolism. Phosphorous MRS can thus be used to measure changes resulting from diseases of muscle cells that involve energy metabolism. Under- or overactivity of some areas of the brain could ultimately be used to warn of a disorder detectable by MRS. After making a diagnosis, the clinician could continue to use MRS to keep an eye on the course of a disease and the effect of drug therapy. MRS has also been used as a research tool, yielding new information on Alzheimer's disease, schizophrenia, autism, stroke, and the normal development and aging of the brain.

One of the latest applications of magnetic signals is in magnetic source imaging, which takes advantage of fact that every discharge of electricity is accompanied by a magnetic field, albeit often a weak one. This technique locates the sources of the very weak fields that accompany the electrical firing of nerve cells in the brain. The extremely sensitive detectors of magnetic source imaging are arranged around the patient's head to track varying levels of activity in many locations of the brain. At present, magnetic source imaging is most effectively used to locate the point of origin of epileptic seizures. Precision is the chief concern here; often, further seizures can be prevented altogether by excision of the tiny area of the brain identified as the focal point. Surrounding areas are able to compensate for any loss of function.

One other imaging technique, ultrasound, has a rather specific application for the brain. A noninvasive technique, like all those discussed here, ultrasound offers the additional advantage that the form of radiation it uses—acoustic waves—is widely agreed to pose virtually no threat of side effects. Ultrasound has become familiar to many women during pregnancy, because it is often used as a means to examine the fetus in the uterus, without adverse effects. The technique works by directing a pulse of acoustic waves at some body structure and then measuring the strength and speed of the waves that bounce off the body and return as echoes. Assuming an average speed for sound waves through body tissues (about 1,540 meters per second), the ultrasound device assembles the various echo times into an image. Organs and connective tissue tend to reflect sound waves quite differently, so that the outline of structures can be seen distinctly. Ultrasound can also produce useful images of blood flow and of structures that are moving, with a fairly high resolution of about 0.5 to 1 millimeter.

Sound waves penetrate very poorly through bone, and this fact might appear to make ultrasound imaging of the brain impossible. However, in one special case—the newborn baby, in whom the bones of the skull are quite thin and have not yet fused together—ultrasound can be invaluable, offering a chance to examine the brain without surgery.

REWARDING COMBINATIONS

Each imaging technique presented in this chapter has its own set of advantages and drawbacks that determine its best applications. For instance, the comparative approach described earlier for panic disorder and depression and their functional equivalents in everyday experience is a way to use the young technology of PET to full advantage. Even more powerful as an aid to research is the combination of PET with other forms of imaging. Although no technique currently available can do justice to the whole picture, each one offers a unique glimpse into the intricacies of the living brain.

ACKNOWLEDGMENT

Chapter 3 is based on presentations by Marcus Raichle.

4

The Role of the Brain in Mental Illness

The brain has not always been esteemed as the locus of that highly complex and contradictory entity, the human mind. In ancient Egypt, the soul and all mental functioning were thought to be located in the heart, although some scholars assigned this role to the liver. Hippocrates, in fourth-century (B.C.) Greece, identified the brain as "the interpreter of consciousness" and deduced that various forms of madness can arise from an unhealthy brain. He also held, though, that the brain was a gland and was most important as the site at which air, with its vital properties, was drawn into the body and entered the blood. Aristotle, for his part, considered the brain merely a cooling organ at the top of the body.

Early Christian thought located mental functions in the ventricles of the brain, along a progression from the front of the head toward the back: sensation and imagination in the anterior ventricle, reason and intellect in the third ventricle, and memory, as the most selective mental faculty, in the rearmost ventricle. In the eighteenth and nineteenth centuries, the popular science of phrenology sought to assign every conceivable trait of personality to its own specific location on the cerebral cortex, as if the mind were a physical entity like the brain. Most recently,

46

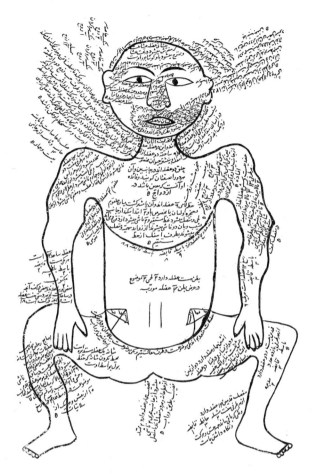

FIGURE 4.1. The medical basis of mental illness was under study as long ago as the fifteenth century, in Persia. This watercolor drawing from an anatomical textbook of 1488 reports beliefs about the correspondences between certain forms of mental illness and particular parts of the body. Source: Tashrih al-badan, 1488. The National Library of Medicine.

neuroscience has begun to uncover some of the intricate and less obvious relations between the mind and the brain, as investigative approaches from biochemistry, psychology, and genetics converge on an understanding of the physiology of mental illness.

In the 1980s, a new willingness to consider disorders of mental functioning as a proper concern of public health, and thus an appropriate field for epidemiological study, led to the first attempt in this country to survey mental health on a national scale. The results, released in 1985 by the National Institute of Mental Health, were startling. Mental illnesses—syndromes and behavioral signs specific enough to be recognized, diagnosed, and, increasingly, treated effectively—are far from rare. On any given day, as extrapolated from the NIMH study population, 12 percent of adults in the United States—more than one in eight—suffer from a mental disorder. The toll is thus exceedingly high: in our collective lifetime, as many as 30 million Americans will at some point endure the disability, pain, and disruption of quality of life that come with a mental disorder. Many more will be touched, of course, through their concern for a family member, friend, or co-worker.

But the news is not all bad. With the efforts of numerous scientific disciplines—the combined approach that is a hallmark of neuroscience—the successes have begun to add up, at first slowly. Current work in the laboratory and in clinical practice builds on the basic research and clinical practice of the past, offering better prospects than before for alleviating a number of mental disorders. Multidisciplinary efforts have also made considerable progress toward untangling the factors at the root of some mental illnesses, bringing closer the goal of early detection or even of prevention to some degree, by interrupting a chain of factors.

MANIC-DEPRESSIVE ILLNESS

One of the better known success stories of this field has been the use of lithium to alleviate manic-depressive disorder. This bipolar illness, with its short phase of gregariousness, seemingly boundless energy, and ambition followed by deadening, slow-moving depression, tends to make its first appearance before the age of 35; the syndrome has been described (by the British psychoanalyst D. W. Winnicott) as "the mania being unreal and the depression being intolerable." Little wonder that, according to public health studies, a manic-depressive patient without effective treatment could expect to spend almost half his or her adult life disabled, either in the hospital or at home grappling with or recovering from a cycle of illness. The use of lithium in controlling this disorder was approved by the Food and Drug Administration in 1969; the benefits, in suffering averted and in recovered productivity, have been enormous. According to one estimate from NIMH, in a little more than 20 years, this use of lithium has saved the United States $39 billion.

Although the impact of lithium on manic-depressive illness is unmistakable, the biochemical means by which it works are not yet well understood. Family studies that examine inherited traits over several generations indicate at least some genetic basis for the illness: in sets of identical twins, if one twin suffers from the disorder, in almost 50 percent of cases the other twin does too. By contrast, the concordance rate in fraternal twins is only about 10 percent, the same as for other siblings. Adopted children have been found to suffer from the illness at a rate more in accord with that of their birth parents than of their adoptive parents, although environment, upbringing, and individual psychological makeup also clearly play a role in developing the illness (if this were not so, pairs of identical twins would tend to be affected in exactly the same way).

Lithium was first used for treating mania in 1948, in Australia, after psychiatrist John Cade observed that it had a calming effect on guinea pigs. The treatment for bipolar disorder nowadays is usually administered in the form of the common salt lithium carbonate; this compound appears to reduce the intensity of both the manic and the depressive phases, producing something of an evening out of mood. Just how the one compound could inhibit both extremes is unclear. One possibility is that as a salt, lithium may affect the passage of charged ions across cell membranes, which are controlled in part by sodium and calcium "gates" (as explained in Chapter 2).

OBSESSIVE-COMPULSIVE DISORDER

Obsessive-compulsive disorder, which had long challenged physicians with its almost limitless variety of forms, is a mental dysfunction that is only beginning to yield to biochemical therapy. Because the patient often is healthy and appears to function capably outside the area of the compulsion, the basis of obsessive-compulsive behavior was thought for some time to be purely psychological, and the favored method of treatment was some form of psychotherapy. Physiological explanations seemed unable to account for the bewildering assortment of symptoms and behavioral tics brought about by this illness—from checking for the twentieth time that the door is locked before going out, to washing one's hands hundreds of times a day, to retracing a driving route yet again to make sure one had really not hit that pedestrian.

Certain drugs or injuries to the head have been known, however, to bring on compulsive behavior. Moreover, family studies show a significant rate of concordance for the illness in identical twins, regardless of whether they are brought up together or separately. Clearly, an explanation of obsessive-compulsive disorder must at least allow room for a physiological factor, traceable in part to the individual's genetic makeup. And yet biology, even molecular biology, cannot give the full picture, because studies of twins have also shown that when both develop the illness, each experiences his or her own obsessions and enacts his or her own distinct compulsions. Most recently, investigators have been able to induce some of the symptoms of obsessive-compulsive disorder in experimental animals. With the identification of an animal model come strong leads for further study, such as selective mating of the animal to trace the genetic patterns in more detail and comparisons of different circumstances for raising the young. Following up these leads should help scientists gain a better idea of how and when a genetic predisposition toward the disorder may be amplified by the environment and to what degree.

On the clinical front, obsessive-compulsive disorder is yielding to treatment with a class of drugs that inhibits the uptake of the neurotransmitter serotonin. One of the most successful of these drugs has been clomipramine, which effectively blocks the uptake of serotonin at synapses; it also affects somewhat the uptake of another neurotransmitter, norepinephrine. In PET scans of patients given clomipramine, activity throughout the cortex and the basal ganglia (involved in the control of movement) is close to normal levels, rather than noticeably higher as is characteristic of obsessive-compulsive disorder. More tangibly, under clomipramine the patient's compulsive acts or rituals abate, sometimes by as much as half. However, while medication can bring relief from the physical symptoms, it leaves untouched the obsessive state of mind that not only calls for the compulsive acts but also makes sense of them, attributing to them some rationale that lets them fit into the patient's world view. Thus both medication and some form of psychological counseling may be needed in the treatment of obsessive-compulsive disorder—truly a mind-brain disease.

PANIC DISORDER

Another malady to come under the scrutiny of neuroscience is panic disorder—a serious disability that has only recently been recognized as such, and whose physiological basis in the brain is just beginning to come to light. Estimated by some researchers to afflict as many as 1.5 million Americans, this disorder makes itself known by sporadic, inexplicable spells of panic: sudden intense feelings of fear and dread, choking or smothering, hyperventilation, irregular heartbeat, and extreme dizziness, together with a sense that one is about to die. Patients may suffer one panic attack a week or several attacks a day. Under this lash, some individuals grow afraid to leave their home; many are heavy users of emergency medical services, forming a large proportion of those mistakenly diagnosed with heart attacks, for example. In addition, the rate of attempted suicide among people with panic disorder is 20 times higher than among the population at large.

A first step toward understanding this illness was a clearcut definition that could be used consistently in studying the disorder from all angles. For example, if a particular compound or class of drugs was found to block panic anxiety specifically and consistently, this response could be used as a criterion for diagnosing the disorder. Certain antidepressant medications appeared indeed to work this way, as did several minor tranquilizers; this combination of effects set panic anxiety apart from less intense chronic anxiety and from transient feelings of panic, states that are unaffected by antidepressant drugs.

Also crucial to a definition, of course, was identifying what triggers panic attacks. The strong consensus of a number of research teams points not to external events or conditions but to chemical factors in the blood. Panic attacks can be brought on by an excess of sodium lactate (like the lactate produced by muscles as a by-product of strenuous exercise), by substances that block the action of the "stress hormone" epinephrine, by at least one compound that facilitates the uptake of serotonin, and by inhalation of high concentrations of carbon dioxide.

At the cellular level, PET scans uncover a striking feature of panic disorder (see Plate 6). During an attack, the brain shows significant asymmetry between the left and right hemispheres, in a region that forms part of the limbic system (the "emotional brain"). In patients with panic disorder, the left side of this region shows lower blood volume and blood flow, and less use of oxygen—in short, less activity. This imbalance is not seen in normal patients, even in conditions of induced anxiety (for instance, when they are told by an experimenter to expect an electric shock), although the *overall* pattern for "normal" anxiety is similar. What distinguishes panic disorder is the asymmetry between the left and right hemispheres and the higher levels of activity overall.

With clear criteria for diagnosis in place, researchers can now pursue new lines of investigation into the origin of the disorder and its mechanism of action in the brain. As with obsessive-compulsive disorder, family studies show a pattern of inheritance—the sign of a genetic factor at work. For panic disorder, the rate of concordance among first-degree relatives is about 15 percent—not terribly high, but still many times the rate at which the illness is found in the general population. Among identical twins the concordance rate is 31 percent. The search is under way for more families touched by this disorder to provide a group of subjects for intensive genetic studies.

As with other important problems in biomedicine, investigating the nature of panic disorder has been fruitful for neuroscience in an unexpected way: it appears that the features of a panic attack can tell us something about the normal brain. In the late 1970s, several laboratory teams produced evidence of some interaction between the receptors for the neurotransmitter known as GABA (gamma-aminobutyric acid) and those for the benzodiazepines, a group of minor tranquilizers. The binding sites for the latter were found to lie close to the GABA receptor sites, as did binding sites for the barbiturates, a class of sedative or hypnotic drugs. The discovery that makes sense of this arrangement is that both the benzodiazepines and the barbiturates work by means of the GABA receptors: they open the chloride ion channel so that negatively charged chloride ions enter the cell. The result is to hyperpolarize the cell membrane, thereby reducing the excitability of the neuron; this brings about a lower level of response to stimuli, which is experienced as a sedating or tranquilizing effect.

This mechanism in turn points back toward panic disorder, in which some patients apparently have a lower than usual sensitivity in their receptors to the benzodiazepines and an increased sensitivity to substances that block the action of those compounds. Animal models of panic disorder all show evidence of abnormality around the hippocampus, where the benzodiazepine-antagonist receptor sites are densely concentrated. Thus, from the perspective both of cell biology and of genetics, a general outline of panic disorder is being filled in with increasing detail.

So far we have considered several illnesses that interfere with the effective functioning of specific cells, usually at the level of chemical signal transmission. Not all mental disorders fall into this category, however. Another category, known as the dementias, arises from progressive degeneration of brain structures. Often, these illnesses pass through several stages of increasing severity.

ALZHEIMER'S DISEASE

Alzheimer's disease is the major form of dementia known in the United States today, affecting an estimated 4 million people. The progressive changes in mental functioning that it causes—disturbances of memory, a lessening ability to take in new information or to coordinate it with what is already known, and sometimes subtle changes in personality—may be slight at first but can soon become most distressing. The toll taken by Alzheimer's is clearly associated with advancing age: it afflicts less than 5 percent of the population below the age of 75, about 20 percent of those aged 75 to 84, and more than 40 percent of

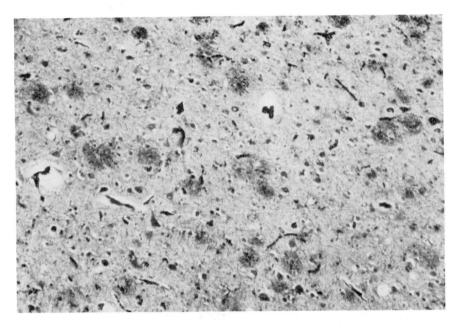

FIGURE 4.2. Tangles of neural fibers and "plaques" in the brain are two of the well-known signs of Alzheimer's disease. The plaques are lesions that contain a protein known as amyloid; their actual role in the course of the disease is still under debate. In this microscopic view of tissue from the cerebral cortex of a patient with Alzheimer's disease, the plaques appear as black knots against the gray background of the more healthy cells. Source: R. Cook-Deegan, taken from archives of the Department of Neurology, University of Colorado.

those aged 85 or older. This profile does not appear to be linked to an American life-style; study populations from various parts of the world have produced similar figures.

Although Alzheimer's disease is widely recognized, the formal criteria for diagnosing it are still under debate. In 1984, a working group of the National Institute of Neurological and Communicative Disorders and Stroke–Alzheimer's Disease and Related Disorders Association, headed by Guy McKhann, director of the Krieger Mind/Brain Institute at Johns Hopkins University, published a report concluding that to diagnose Alzheimer's disease with confidence, the physician should rely on specific signs in the brain. Chief among these were tangled knots of fine neural fibers and so-called "senile plaques," actually microscopic lesions in the brain that contain a starchlike protein known as amyloid.

But McKhann is no longer satisfied with the conclusions of the report, which he now considers "rather myopic"—that is, too closely focused on the visible pathology of plaques and tangles. He believes instead that what is called Alzheimer's disease may not be a single entity at all and that using this simple name may in fact limit the thinking of some researchers, implying as it does that what is sought is the identity of a single disease-causing mechanism. An alternative explanation of the same clinical observations may be that several regions of the nervous system are involved, each one vulnerable to different factors. Combinations of these factors at work could give a clinical picture that is sufficiently similar, enough of the time, to hold together under the heading of Alzheimer's disease.

In the end stage of Alzheimer's, perhaps 5 to 10 years after the onset of disease, the brain shows some degeneration of the frontal and temporal lobes, particularly in the hippocampus, an area involved in short-term memory. Medical imaging reveals a significant loss of neurons, and an even greater loss of synapses—which may provide a better explanation for dementia than the tangles and plaques do. For that matter, the question of what causes dementia has any number of possible answers, most of them exceedingly difficult to disprove. There is even the possibility that such features as loss of short-term memory and reduced ability to learn are just a variant of normal aging. After all, the affected portion of the population forms a steady upward curve on epidemiological graphs. Perhaps everyone would eventually suffer dementia if they lived long enough. Since this theory is not provable, however, it is well to consider other possible causes of dementia. Among those suggested recently have been excitatory amino acids that exert a harmful effect, some form of infectious slow virus, the presence of toxic metals in the brain, vascular disease, time-delayed genetic programming, or some combination of these factors.

Excitatory amino acids can indeed cause severe deficits in the brain, including loss of memory. A dramatic illustration came recently from eastern Canada, where a number of people became seriously ill after eating contaminated mussels. Several died; those who recovered sustained a major loss of memory. Brain scans from some of the victims showed an overwhelming loss of neurons from the hippocampus, similar to the pathology of the substantia nigra (a region involved in the control of movement) seen in Parkinson's disease. The toxin from the mussels proved to be similar to glutamic acid, an excitatory neurotransmitter that occurs naturally in the central nervous system; it was also both highly potent and specific for those regions of the brain that process new memories. Such a substance is under study as a possible agent of Alzheimer's disease, as is the hypothesis that the disorder may be caused by a slow virus. Experimental testing of the virus theory would have to include a demonstrated ability to bring about recognizable "dementia" in laboratory animals solely by infection with the viral agent. Early claims of infection-induced dementia from one laboratory have not yet been replicated, despite attempts by the original group and a number of other research teams.

The theory that the presence of metal in the brain—specifically, aluminum—produces a toxic effect attracted lively interest when it was first advanced in the early 1970s. Evidence of aluminum in the neural tangles was plentiful and striking, and the theory circulated widely, to the point that the public began to wonder about the prudence of using aluminum cookware, for example. However, in the absence of evidence that further supports this theory or suggests how aluminum may work its harmful effects, the metal has lost some of its prominence as a possible cause of Alzheimer's. A current interpretation proposes instead that the aluminum in neural tangles may be a secondary effect, whose role (if any) in the development of this disease is unclear. Aluminum is, after all, an abundant element on earth, occurring naturally in water, soil, and much of our plant and animal food. Its presence in the brain may actually be the result of cells dying, rather than the cause; but this point is still under debate.

Vascular disease may figure in the onset of some dementias. The hippocampus is known to be an area of the brain that is highly susceptible to changes in blood flow; thus, some disruption of vascular function is being considered as at least a factor in the deficits of memory and new learning that characterize Alzheimer's, if not the primary factor. The question that would remain, of course, is what gives rise to the vascular disease that causes these disabilities.

Genetic factors currently offer an exciting line of research into Alzheimer's disease. Recent success in locating the genetic region for another degenerative neurological disease, Huntington's chorea, has fostered the hope of a similar discovery for Alzheimer's. It appears that some families may have a gene on chromosome 21 that is associated with Alzheimer's disease. Another group of families among whom the disease develops later in life may have an affected gene on chromosome 19. Still other families in which Alzheimer's disease appears to be genetically based, however, show no evidence of an association with either chromosome. It seems likely that more than one gene can cause Alzheimer's disease, and the number of cases that are mainly genetic in origin remains uncertain.

A different sort of genetic lead comes from the observation that Down's syndrome, which is known to be caused by a mutation of chromosome 21, takes the form of mental retardation followed by dementia. The specific mutation is the existence of three chromosomes (or three copies of part of the chromosome) instead of the usual two, but the molecular biological mechanisms by which this surplus affects mental functioning are not yet understood.

An added reason to look at chromosome 21 is that the gene that codes for amyloid—the protein contained in senile plaques—is located there. Affected patients in a few families with Alzheimer's disease have shown a consistent defect in their amyloid gene. The normal aging human brain also contains amyloid, and the walls of blood vessels bear a similar material; some researchers have suggested therefore that the amyloid found in plaques is transported there from other, "healthy" sites. The mechanism for this process, which would involve a defect in the breakdown of amyloid from a larger precursor molecule, is under investigation by Dennis Selkoe, of the Harvard Medical School, and others.

Another explanation proposes that the low levels of acetylcholine observed in Alzheimer's disease could be an analogue to the low levels of another neurotransmitter, dopamine, observed in Parkinson's disease. According to this rationale, methods of treatment that increase acetylcholine to normal levels should halt the degeneration and loss of neurons. (Acetylcholine can be increased by administering precursors of the neurotransmitter, which the patient's system then breaks down in a normal way, or by blocking the destruction of acetylcholine so that it is active longer.) In addition, several other neurotransmitters clearly suffer some deficit in Alzheimer's disease, so that multiple replacement of neurotransmitters, or the use of drugs that act like transmitters, are options for treatment that should be examined.

The administration of nerve growth factor has been a newsworthy step in laboratory attempts to prevent degeneration of the nerve fiber tracts known as the cholinergic pathways. In animals, nerve growth factor successfully protects the neurons of the hippocampus from dying, which should in turn preserve the workings of short-term memory. But applying such a therapy to humans raises several practical questions: how might a large molecule like nerve growth factor be made to cross the blood-brain barrier, and how would it then be directed to the specific region of the brain where it is needed? Two proposed solutions are a form of reservoir or pump implanted in the brain to give a continuous infusion of the compound, and the use of smaller molecules—analogues of nerve growth factor—that might pass more easily throughout the brain to the required sites. Preliminary reports of the use of nerve growth factor in a small trial, which have appeared recently, are exciting, but they have not yet been confirmed.

Meanwhile, stepping back to the perspective of epidemiology, researchers have posed a fruitful question by turning the usual query about dementia into its opposite. In other words, who does *not* get dementia? What are the factors that allow someone to reach an advanced age and continue to function successfully? For now, both this angle of investigation and the straightforward inquiry into agents of disease call for more and better understood study populations. In long-lived Americans it is especially difficult to sort out the factors that may have affected health over the course of, say, 80 years; however, studies in some regions of the world that have changed less rapidly than this country may be able to assemble populations that show less variability—both among individuals and throughout the life-span.

The prospects for a thorough understanding of Alzheimer's disease are good. After an initial stage during which there appeared to be almost too much information, research from various branches of neuroscience should settle into a coherent picture that will be both satisfying in theory and applicable in clinical practice. Further work in this area will continue to be shaped by advances elsewhere in neuroscience and, at the same time, is well situated to help impel those advances.

Three areas of particular interest are the mechanisms at the cellular level that enable learning and memory (see Chapter 7), a clearer understanding of how Alzheimer's disease acts in the brain at each stage, and ways to protect specific regions of the nervous system from damage or perhaps even to reverse damage. Another advance in epidemiology would be to gather study populations whose health factors are thoroughly known and homogeneous, to address satisfactorily the two-sided question of what brings on dementia with increasing age and what permits increasing age without dementia. Many specialists in this area feel that the current position of research on Alzheimer's disease resembles that of work on Parkinson's disease about 15 years ago, when the cause and some effective therapies were just about to come to light. Now, with the course of this disease broadly understood and the therapies continuing to improve, Parkinson's is on its way to becoming a manageable disease. The mood is hopeful that Alzheimer's will follow suit.

AIDS-RELATED DEMENTIA

Not all dementias take a steady toll, like Alzheimer's, largely from among the elderly. One form that is spreading through a mixed-age population, on the basis of different risk factors altogether, is AIDS-related dementia (see Plate 2).

Human immunodeficiency virus (HIV) was established as the cause of AIDS in 1983. In 1985 it was recognized as a lentivirus—that is, a virus that primarily infects the macrophages and leads to multisystem chronic disease, including encephalitis (inflammation of the brain). By 1986, it was clear that infection of the nervous system was to be a major feature of AIDS. (Indeed, an HIV-positive but otherwise healthy individual who develops dementia can now be diagnosed, on the basis of that one symptom alone, as having AIDS.) What was not yet clear in 1986 was *when* the infections of the brain and nervous system were taking place, and whether they could be expected in most AIDS cases, given enough time. In other words, do infections of the brain and nervous system form an inherent stage in the course of AIDS in an individual, or should they be considered instead under the heading of the many opportunistic infections that attack the hobbled immune system in late-stage AIDS?

Questions of this degree of complexity call for the long-term cooperation of a consistent population of volunteers. In 1985 the Multicenter AIDS Cohort Study (MACS) recruited 480 homosexual and bisexual men into a cohort that included individuals who were HIV positive, some who seroconverted (that is, their blood began to test positive for HIV) at some point during the study, and others who remained HIV negative and served as control subjects. At the beginning, the study involved psychological testing and neurological examination; a smaller group underwent nuclear magnetic resonance imaging, electroencephalography, and a spinal tap at regular intervals, and they continue to volunteer for these painful and arduous tests as investigations proceed today with this same cohort.

The conclusions of this early component of the study were that infection of the nervous system occurs in most cases, and that it takes place quite early—perhaps even at the time of seroconversion, although the infected person may not suffer any symptoms for a considerable time. As to which infections are intrinsic to AIDS and which are opportunistic, the picture is still incomplete. Many diseases of the nervous system are known to be associated with the human immunodeficiency virus; some strike early in the course of infection and some later, when the patient's immune system is gravely suppressed. The diseases range from common to very rare, and they differ in their pathology: some destroy the myelin sheath that protects nerve fibers, others harm the axon or cause gradual loss of nerve cells. This broad variation suggests that the diseases work by means of different biological mechanisms and that a unifying explanation will not be easy to piece together.

A close look at AIDS-related dementia raises questions that apply to other diseases as well. Dementia is found at increasing rates throughout the course of AIDS infection: from about 3 percent at the time that AIDS is first diagnosed to 8–16 percent of HIV-positive outpatients at a hospital clinic, to more than 60 percent of AIDS patients at the time of death. In theory, the prevalence of AIDS-related dementia could be even higher; some specialists estimate that the pathology that underlies it is present in 90 percent of terminal AIDS cases. This observation appears to point toward some form of slow dementia, which incubates over a period of 5 to 10 years and eventually affects cognitive function. Most long-term studies so far suggest that even if the brain is infected early, neuropsychological processes continue unimpaired up to a late stage.

The physical signs of disease in the brain that can be gleaned from medical imaging are also quite subtle up to a late stage of the disease, as reported by Richard T. Johnson, director of the neurology department at Johns Hopkins Medical School. Close examination of the tissues of the brain reveals some frayed white matter, often containing macrophages, and occasionally an abnormally large cell that appears to contain viral antigen, but in general no striking appearance of disease. The pathology is also evident in the spinal cord; here, one finds many macrophages, some demyelination, and, curiously, at the same time some remyelination or resheathing of nerve fibers. The virus itself is thought to reside largely in the macrophages and in microglia, cells that develop from macrophages and whose function in the brain is unclear.

The features of AIDS-related dementia actually correlate best with a demyelinating disease, and, in fact, demyelination has been observed to some degree. The means by which it comes about, however, are still unclear. One promising line of study focuses on cytokines, which, like antibodies, are a product of the immune system. It appears that the infection may induce a particular cytokine to attack the myelin sheaths; this possibility is under examination. Another question is whether the viral proteins, those contained in the macrophages, for example, are toxic to cells or are harmful because they block the access of neurotransmitters to cells. Another possibility is transactivation, in which a gene from the AIDS virus acts as the "on" switch for a genetic sequence outside itself—either in neural cells of the human host or in another virus infecting the patient at the same time. At present, opportunistic infections do not appear to be the agent of AIDS-related dementia; consequently, research is aimed toward deciphering the steps by which dementia could be produced by the AIDS virus itself. The major impact of the virus, according to scientific consensus, falls on T-4 cells, the "helper cells" of the immune system, and on monocytes, which later develop into macrophages. The monocyte is thought to be the essential cell that figures in the long incubation period between infection and the onset of disease; it may be that monocytes eventually enter the brain as infected macrophages, or they may infect macrophages already in the brain and cause them to release a substance injurious to the nerve cells.

The challenge of AIDS grows more pressing as the virus continues to spread and as more people infected several years ago reach later stages of disease. By current estimates, 1 to 2 million people in the United States are HIV positive; the figure worldwide is more than 5 million. One hopeful finding is that the neuropsychological damage, fairly early on, responds well to treatment with zidovudine, or AZT. That the dementia is reversible, even if only to a limited extent, bodes well for the future therapy of a debilitating disease. Meanwhile, it is crucial to widen the research perspective to include populations that have been neglected thus far and that bring their own factors to the epidemiological formula. For example, what are the special health risks associated with the AIDS virus in intravenous drug users or the ways the virus affects women differently from men or children differently from adults? Research in this field has taken shape quickly, moving in less than 10 years from the earliest observations of nervous system disease to focused molecular biological studies of the disease-causing virus.

DISORDERS OF MOOD AND MIND

To an observer of neuroscience, it is remarkable how permeable are the borders between the brain and the mind when both are considered as objects of study. There is a paradox worth pointing out here, although it is well beyond the scope of this book to explore it: the more neuroscience devotes its attention to obtaining a thorough physiological account of what the brain is doing on a minute molecular level, the more the research tends to find itself in the realm of the psychological, offering information of an entirely different order than what had previously been understood about compulsive behavior, about panic, even about extremes of mood. Successful integration of the two forms of knowledge will provide the most help to patients of mental disorders, as well as, ultimately, yielding the most satisfying explanations. Such coordinated accounts of mental illness are being worked out for many disorders. Even chronic depression, which may be experienced entirely as a response of mood and mind to external events, has its biochemical side.

Observations from a variety of studies of depression have begun to fit together. For one thing, a handful of medications have proved to be effective in treating this disorder—so much so that they are now specifically called the antidepressants—and all of these seem to work by raising the brain's available levels of the same two neurotransmitters, serotonin and norepinephrine. For another thing, information about the drug reserpine has added to the base of knowledge. Once prescribed for high blood pressure, reserpine brought about depression as an unwanted side effect in about 15 percent of cases: in correcting hypertension, it reduced the levels of serotonin and norepinephrine available at the synaptic cleft. More recent studies seem to show that the receptors for at least one of these neurotransmitters, norepinephrine, grow less sensitive in depression; but whether this effect is instead of, or in addition to, a lower level of available neurotransmitter is not yet clear. Nor has it been established that the biochemical factors lead to or in any sense cause the drop in mood, energy, motivation, or enjoyment that characterizes depression. Several drugs that are effective in treating depression apparently act by influencing, in different ways, the levels of norepinephrine and serotonin available to receptors. The research into depression may be a good opportunity for obtaining some information on how a disorder that is experienced mainly in the mind can bring about its own chemical changes in the brain.

SCHIZOPHRENIA

The investigation of schizophrenia is a challenge of quite another kind. Here, there seem to be almost too many factors, and too many markers or manifestations. Schizophrenia is named for the abnormal division or split ("schizo") between thought and emotion that characterizes the disorder in many cases. Striking about 1 percent of the population, schizophrenia can bring hallucinations, delusions, and profound withdrawal from normal social or family contact. An episode of schizophrenia can pass off spontaneously, but many individuals struggle for years in a snare of imagined scenes and voices, paranoia, and self-isolation, all of which reinforce one another. Patients suffering from schizophrenia number more than 1 million in the United States and occupy more than 100,000 hospital beds on any given day. As with so many mental disorders, the toll is unacceptably high; yet effective means of intervention or, ideally, of prediction and prevention have been largely out of reach while the illness itself is incompletely understood.

In the 1950s, a medication called chlorpromazine was found to reduce some of the more troubling symptoms, such as hallucinations and imagined voices. Although it did not address the delusional thinking that can come to shape the patient's whole world view in a case of chronic schizophrenia, its relief of overt symptoms promised to make life at least a little more manageable for many schizophrenic patients, and, in the 1960s, thousands were released from institutional care on the strength of that promise. But, although chlorpromazine offered relief from some symptoms, it could not cure the underlying disease.

It has remained for later decades to begin to unravel several lines of evidence about the nature of schizophrenia. Chlorpromazine, as well as several other drugs that relieve schizophrenic symptoms, works by blocking the brain's receptor sites for dopamine, particularly in the prefrontal cortex. More specifically, experiments at the National Institute of Mental Health and in Scandinavia in which schizophrenic patients were asked to perform cognitive tasks showed that these individuals have abnormally low activity in that area of the brain.

Such findings give rise to speculation about just what goes

on in the prefrontal cortex. It has been suggested that this area of the brain is concerned with the process of working memory, which underlies the ability to regulate behavior by ideas and concepts. For instance, Patricia Goldman-Rakic, professor of neuroscience at Yale University School of Medicine, has found that rhesus monkeys with lesions in the prefrontal cortex are unable to hold information "in mind" for even a few seconds; their behavior is erratic, distracted, and meaninglessly repetitive. They are also unable to follow a fast-moving target with their eyes, although their ability to follow a slow-moving target is unimpaired. Altogether, these deficits mimic some of the signs of schizophrenia. They also point to a defect in information processing: the loss of a capacity to predict where the target will be in the next fraction of a second, or the loss of ability to predict events in general.

It may appear unreasonable at first to single out one specific area of the brain to account for a disorder as global and wide ranging in its symptoms as schizophrenia. (Indeed, this area may well prove to be only one region out of many that play a role.) Still, its involvement seems plausible when we consider that the prefrontal cortex occupies one-quarter of the entire cerebral cortex and interconnects with many other regions and with the limbic system—including some areas that show evidence for related dysfunction in cases of schizophrenia. Disorders of the senses (hallucinations) and sudden urgent feelings of anger or fear can all be traced, at least in neurophysiological theory, to misfiring synapses in one area or another of the sensory association cortex or of the limbic system, which controls mood. Another point in favor of this line of thinking is that the frontal lobe contains the highest concentration of dopamine fibers in the cerebrum, and the specific dopamine receptor that is the primary site of action of antipsychotic drugs is known to reside in this area. Thus, a biological explanation for schizophrenia is beginning to evolve. It remains true, however, that the particulars of any case, the form of the hallucinations and delusions in an individual's mind, can only be approached in psychological terms. Similarly, although dopamine blockers may relieve the brain somewhat of symptoms, psychosocial therapy can dramatically help the patient in day-today living, by offering the chance to improve coping skills: how to remember to take medications reliably, how to manage in stressful situations, how to interact socially with others.

Research on schizophrenia has also brought neuroscientists a step closer to an understanding of how the prefrontal cortex functions in normal circumstances. Current scientific thinking is that the region guides behavior by its representations, or working memory, of stimuli rather than by direct perception of the stimuli themselves. (Hence the inability in schizophrenia to predict the location of a moving target or to foresee an expectable outcome in given circumstances, for instance, in social interactions.) In a general sense it can be said that this area of the brain—which is greatly enlarged in humans, relative to our near-cousins, the other primates—provides the physiological basis for abstract thought and the ability to plan.

Vigorous investigation into the many forms and factors of mental illness is thus a central task for neuroscience. Observations from clinical practice, laboratory study of the mechanisms of disease and the ability of chemical compounds to harm or help, and genetic analysis of family history all build on one another, offering the prospect of more efficacious treatments and of theoretical accounts that grow more solid as new details are filled in. While neuroscience looks more closely at the brain, it continues to enlarge our options for treating the mind.

ACKNOWLEDGMENTS

Chapter 4 is based on presentations by Patricia Goldman-Rakic, Richard Johnson, Lewis Judd, and Guy McKhann.

5

From Chemistry to Circuitry

In an uncanny way, the images of everyday speech can sometimes anticipate formal scientific knowledge. Who at one time or another has not compared an idea to an electrical spark or spoken of the "chemistry" of a particular mood? The brain does indeed convey its signals by means of electricity and chemical compounds; so much is well known. But the finer details of how it actually manages these transmissions, and at prodigious speeds—sometimes firing several hundred nerve impulses in a second—still make for fascinating inquiry.

The scientific understanding of electricity in the nervous system has come a long way since the 1700s, when Luigi Galvani of Bologna noticed that disembodied frog legs hanging on copper hooks from an iron balcony would occasionally twitch, as if still animated. On the basis of this observation and subsequent experiments, he concluded that the motive force in the nervous system was electricity rather than the traditionally conceived "animal spirits." Galvani could scarcely have imagined the bacterial robots, electron diffraction microscopes, and positron emission tomography devices that would come to replace the accoutrements of an eighteenth-century Italian kitchen as the proper equipment for scientific observation. And he would be

68

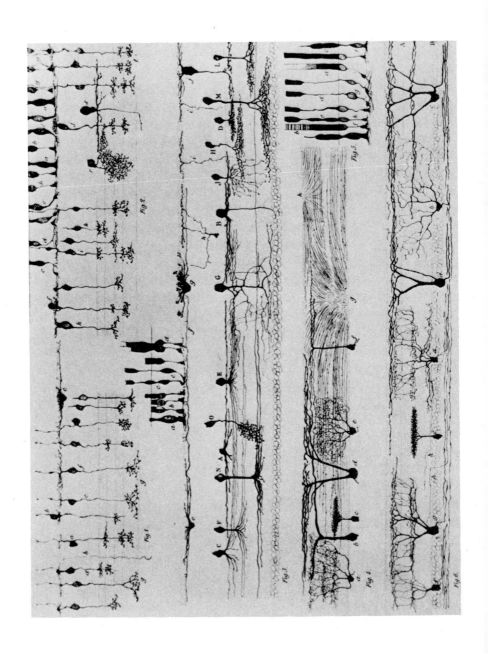

equally astonished by today's cogent, nearly molecule-by-molecule explanation of just what was twitching in those frog legs.

CHEMICALS AS SIGNALS

Unlike electricity, the brain's chemical messengers, the neurotransmitters, are difficult to identify from first observations. The action of electricity could be confirmed or disproved by home-style tests; but the activity and nature of a chemical compound that may be involved in the brain's signaling system demand more rigorous examination. The compound must meet a half dozen specific criteria to be considered a neurotransmitter—as opposed to, say, a "second messenger" in the brain, which broadcasts signals within a cell rather than conveying a signal from one cell to another. (Distinctions such as this, which may seem overly fine at first, have a way of turning out later to be crucial for understanding new, otherwise inexplicable data.)

To be recognized as a neurotransmitter, a chemical compound must satisfy six conditions: It must be (1) synthesized in the neuron, (2) stored there, and (3) released in sufficient quantity to bring about some physical effect; (4) when administered experimentally, the compound must demonstrate the same effect that it brings about in living tissue; and (5) there must be receptor sites specific to this compound on the postsynaptic membrane, as well as (6) a means for shutting off its effect, either by causing its swift decomposition or by reuptake, absorbing it back into the cell. Of course, before any of these items on the checklist come into question, the compound must somehow be detectable in the human brain—not always an easy matter, in view of the minute quantities involved.

One of the first substances to pass all the tests was acetylcholine (ACh). Widespread throughout the central nervous system, ACh usually has an excitatory function, but it can also

FIGURE 5.1. Pen-and-ink drawings were the first scientific illustrations to depict the actual structure of individual nerve cells. Several types of neurons are represented here; each has a recognizably thicker portion that is the cell body, and most have a single axon that projects like a thin wire. The number and the branching patterns of each cell's dendrites show more variation. Source: D. Santiago Ramón y Cajal, 1889. *Manuel de Histología Normal y Técnica Micrográphia*. The National Library of Medicine.

be inhibitory, depending on prevailing conditions at the receptor site. Because ACh acts briskly and is subject to prompt breakdown in the synaptic cleft, it is well suited as the transmitter for motor neurons. Acetylcholine also acts in the autonomic nervous system, where it is responsible for such functions as contracting the pupil of the eye, slowing heartbeat, and stimulating salivation and digestion.

Two poisons that are well known to readers of mystery novels work their deadly effects by blocking the action of ACh. Curare, a plant extract used by South American Indians to treat their arrows for hunting, rapidly causes paralysis; botulin, a toxin produced by bacteria in improperly canned foods, paralyzes the muscles that control breathing and thereby causes suffocation. In clinical practice, drugs that block the action of ACh are useful in many ways. Short-lived ACh inhibitors are given in eye drops to dilate the pupil for ophthalmic examination. More enduring forms, such as atropine, reduce the secretion of saliva and bronchial fluid, which is helpful for anesthesia; hyoscine, or scopolamine, another related compound, is sometimes used as a sedative but does have the side effect of causing a very dry mouth. Conversely, drugs that inhibit the chemical breakdown of ACh and thus extend its action in the synaptic cleft are at least temporarily effective against myasthenia gravis; this is a crippling disease in which the body's own immune system attacks the receptor sites for ACh on the skeletal muscles. The muscles gradually weaken as they receive fewer synaptic transmissions, but drugs such as eserine can effectively increase the amount of ACh available to the remaining receptor sites.

In the cerebral cortex, ACh is thought to play a role in storing short-term memories. The hippocampus, for example, has dense areas of receptor sites for ACh, and their degeneration is one of the biological signs of Alzheimer's disease (see Chapter 4). Thus far, attempts to reverse symptoms by giving drugs that mimic or enhance the action of ACh have not been successful.

Along with ACh, another transmitter that is widely encountered throughout the nervous system is norepinephrine (also known as noradrenaline). In the central nervous system, the function of norepinephrine usually complements that of ACh; thus norepinephrine acts in the general direction of arousal, and ACh tends toward restorative functions. Norepinephrine dilates the pupil of the eye, strengthens and speeds the heartbeat, and inhibits processes of digestion, all under the heading of what has been called the "fight or flight" response; it also stimulates the adrenal glands to release epinephrine and the liver to release large quantities of glucose, which make more energy available to the muscles for action. Several drugs that work by means of the norepinephrine system are useful in asthma; these are known as the beta-agonists, because they are targeted to a specific group of "beta" receptors in the bronchial muscles, where they relieve constriction.

In some instances, norepinephrine may function not as a transmitter but as a neuromodulator, promoting or blocking the action of some other transmitter at the synapse. Experimental evidence on this point is still coming in; if the hypothesis holds up, it would add a new detail to an already crowded picture and could open up other lines of investigation as well.

The neurons in the brain that contain norepinephrine cluster in a small region of the brainstem; their axons project to the hypothalamus, the cerebellum, and even the forebrain, a good 10 to 15 centimeters away. Norepinephrine is associated not only with alertness and arousal but also with the dreaming phase of sleep and, by way of the hypothalamus and the limbic system, with the regulation of mood. For instance, a number of studies point to depleted levels of norepinephrine at brain synapses, or a reduced ability of receptors to use it, as a factor in depression. Not that this amounts to a scientific formula that a normal brain minus some amount of norepinephrine equals a depressed mind; such formulas are far too coarse—particularly in an area like the basis of mood, where any number of elements may interact. Moreover, some of the factors that are undoubtedly important for mood are unquantifiable, invisible, and perhaps irreproducible for laboratory study. One point of wide consensus, however, is that depression can be helped by two classes of drugs: one class blocks an enzyme that would normally break down norepinephrine in the synaptic cleft, and the other slows the reuptake of norepinephrine into the presynaptic cell.

The neurotransmitter serotonin is a powerful constrictor of

blood flow and an inhibitor of some sensations of pain; in recent years, its intriguing variety of effects on our mental life have also come under study. Serotonin is of great importance in regulating sleep; the old folk remedy for sleeplessness, a glass of warm milk before bedtime, may work because of the presence in milk of tryptophan, an amino acid that the brain uses to make serotonin.

This transmitter can affect many parts of the brain at once through the long-reaching axons of serotonergic (serotonin-using) neurons, which underlie the transmitter's role in such global phenomena as sleep and mood. The drugs that raise levels of available norepinephrine to alleviate depression also work on serotonin, by the same mechanisms. (Interestingly, the axons that carry serotonin are not myelinated. Without the electrical insulation afforded by the myelin sheath, impulses travel at less than the lightning speed achieved by, say, signals to the motor neurons, but this seems appropriate to the more global and subjective areas of life regulated by serotonin.) The remarkable effects of lysergic acid diethylamide, or LSD, in even the tiniest quantities, are based on its strong chemical resemblance to serotonin; it is as if a full system of preexisting receptor sites lies ready for the drug's use.

One further aspect of this versatile transmitter is that serotonin is featured in biochemical accounts of "sensitization," the enhanced response to a stimulus as a result of training. Scientists have studied sensitization in extraordinary detail in simple animals such as the marine snail as a model for more complex processes of learning in the human brain (see Chapter 7).

Dopamine is chemically similar to serotonin and norepinephrine, and it overlaps with them in several biological functions. Formed, like serotonin, from an amino acid, dopamine is actually a precursor to norepinephrine—the same compound except for one different chemical bond—and a wide-ranging neurotransmitter in its own right. In many systems, dopamine acts as an "off" switch: it halts the release of prolactin (which is responsible for the function of the mammary glands), inhibits some cells of the olfactory tract, and also shuts off some of the action of autonomic nerve cells (although this function is not well understood).

Elsewhere in the nervous system, dopamine is important

for the control of movement; the degeneration of dopamine-using neurons in a portion of the midbrain leads to Parkinson's disease. A patient with this condition finds it difficult to initiate movement and also to stop, and to manage associated actions such as swinging the arms while walking. A slow tremor of the hands and head, present when the patient is at rest but not during movement, is probably what gave the illness its original name of "the shaking palsy." Although the progress of the disease cannot be halted, the symptoms of Parkinson's disease can be effectively controlled in most patients by treatment with L-dopa. (This is not the actual transmitter itself but a precursor, a molecule that has the ability to pass through the blood–brain barrier and from which the brain can form dopamine.)

Because dopaminergic neurons are also well distributed in the limbic system, we would expect some role for this neurotransmitter in the creation of mood—and, indeed, evidence to this effect is accumulating. Most striking are the signs that a relative increase in dopamine activity in the frontal cortex may provide the biochemical basis for schizophrenia.

Evidence for the role of dopamine has come from several directions. Chlorpromazine, a drug first used widely in mental hospitals in the 1950s and 1960s to reduce the overt symptoms of schizophrenia, was found in the 1970s to block the action of dopamine at receptor sites. Then, too, some of the patients who were given the medication to help control their hallucinations and thought disorders developed, over the long term, a tremor and other physical symptoms that resembled those of Parkinson's disease. A third clue may be the ability of amphetamines, when taken in sufficient quantity, to bring on disturbances of the mind much like schizophrenia; it is known that amphetamines, or "uppers," increase the levels of dopamine available in the brain.

To be sure, an illness as complex as schizophrenia cannot be reduced to a simple chemical explanation such as "excess of dopamine." The question remains open whether the schizophrenic brain suffers from too much dopamine, too many dopamine receptors, a standard quantity of receptors with abnormally high sensitivity, or some other dysfunction entirely—to say nothing of the important genetic, social, and psychological factors also under study. Science has a long way to go yet in explaining schizophrenia, and it seems likely that a complete account of the functions of dopamine in the brain may also take some time to fall into place.

Another major neurotransmitter derived from an amino acid is gamma-aminobutyric acid, or GABA. Unlike dopamine or serotonin, which have diverse roles, GABA consistently acts as an "off" signal; the cerebellum, retina, and spinal cord all use this transmitter to inhibit signals, as do many other parts of the brain and nervous system. GABA's inhibitory effect comes about in the following way: the transmitter opens a channel in the membrane through which negatively charged chloride ions can enter the cell. This influx hyperpolarizes the cell and makes it less likely to be excited by incoming stimuli.

GABA receptor sites show some tendency to bind barbiturates and the "minor tranquilizers," the benzodiazepines. Curiously, the presence of GABA in low concentrations enhances the binding of benzodiazepines to receptor sites. This pattern indicates that GABA and the benzodiazepines cannot be competing for exactly the same sites. Instead, an array of recent studies have yielded the view that the GABA receptor site is in fact a multifunctional set of proteins that contain the chloride ion channel and distinct subsites for binding of benzodiazepines, other tranquilizers such as barbiturates, and GABA itself.

RECEPTORS PLAY AN ACTIVE PART

The neurotransmitters discussed thus far are just a few of the ones that have been known for a relatively long time (at least a decade or two). But likely additions to the list number at least 40, and new candidates continue to appear. Even from this brief survey, however, a curious fact emerges: a single neurotransmitter can be responsible for many different effects.

How can a chemical compound, unchanging in various parts of the body or brain, produce diverse results? The answer lies on the other side of the synapse in the receptor sites, which do change their properties to a surprising degree and in the end determine what effect a neurotransmitter has on a cell.

For example, it is by means of different receptors that norepinephrine, which supplies blood vessels in both skeletal muscle and skin, can cause constriction in the vessels of the skin and dilation in those of muscle. As another example, ACh's effect of constricting skeletal muscle cells can be blocked by curare but not by atropine, although the two alkaloids are in some ways similar; in smooth muscles of the intestine, however, the action of ACh can be blocked by atropine but is unaffected by curare. Clearly, the receptor molecules in the two locations have somewhat different shapes, despite their both being devised to respond to ACh.

Acetylcholine also serves to illustrate another level of complexity in the brain's signaling system. In muscle cells, it acts directly, moving positively charged sodium ions into the cell and depolarizing it. In the brain, however, this transmitter works in tandem with a "second messenger," which conveys the signal inside the cell, sometimes amplifying it greatly in the process. (In this sense, the neurotransmitter that traverses the synapse is the "first messenger," although this term is rarely used.)

To date, researchers have identified only two second-messenger systems—which is perhaps just as well for those who wish to understand neurophysiology, because the other kinds of messenger systems identified in the brain are proliferating so rapidly. One system uses the small molecule cyclic adenosine monophosphate (cyclic AMP) as its second messenger; the other system uses the even smaller calcium ion (Ca^{2+}) and two compounds made up partly from the cell membrane itself: inositol triphosphate (IP_3) and diacylglycerol (DG).

Both second-messenger systems have the same goal: to bring about a change in the shape of proteins inside the cell, which either enables or halts such activities as contraction (in a muscle cell, for example) or secretion (in a glandular cell). And both second-messenger systems begin in the same way: the receptor site at the cell membrane surface activates one of the so-called G-proteins (which require guanosine triphosphate to carry out their function). The G-protein in turn activates an enzyme within the membrane, causing a chemical reaction that assembles the second-messenger molecules from precursor molecules available inside the cell. Here the two systems diverge: in one, the enzyme adenylate cyclase removes two phosphate groups from adenosine triphosphate (incidentally releasing energy to the cell) and converts it into cyclic AMP. In the other system, the enzyme phospholipase C cleaves a large lipid molecule into two parts, DG and IP_3 (again, releasing energy in the process).

The second messenger, in the form of many thousands of newly created molecules, is thus in a good position to amplify the signal of a neurotransmitter and to broadcast its message speedily throughout the cell. The second messenger may act directly—by simply binding to a cellular protein and thus changing its structure—or indirectly, by activating another enzyme called a protein kinase, which changes a protein's structure and electrical charge by adding a phosphate group to it. In either case, the result is a change in the shape of the protein and consequently a shift in the activities of the cell. Because of the great potential for amplifying the signal at each step (from first messenger to enzyme to cyclic AMP to protein kinase to phosphorylated protein to switched-on function), just a few molecules of a neurotransmitter can cause target cells to produce several million molecules of a reaction substance in far less time than it takes to read about it.

Of course, signals are propagated even more rapidly when the neurotransmitter works without a second messenger. In contrast, the second-messenger routes of transmission generally lead to effects that are longer lasting.

THE BRAIN'S OWN PAINKILLERS

The identification and study of neurotransmitters is still a very young field that tends to grow in spurts—for example, in the 1970s, when researchers seeking to understand the action of opium-based drugs discovered the existence of an entire system of "natural painkillers" produced by the body itself. These neurotransmitters, known as endorphins, for "endogenous morphine-like substances," reduce the body's sensation of pain and, according to some studies, may also play a role in managing stress. Their release, along with epinephrine, in moments of emergency, shock, or injury could help to explain the apparently unnatural feelings of calm and obliviousness to discomfort that are often reported on such occasions.

For investigators on the trail of these natural painkillers, the first clue was the well-known effectiveness of opiates, which are derived from the juice of the opium poppy. Morphine, in particular, has been used for centuries to relieve pain and bring about a sense of well-being. Heroin, a more concentrated form of poppy juice, produces more intense euphoria and is, in addition, quickly addictive—another clue that these drugs must be working by means of some direct pathway in the brain. Researchers devised a way to test this hypothesis by treating rats with opium derivatives that had been "labeled" with radioactive isotopes. The resultant images showed where the opiates had settled in the brain—in other words, they amounted to a map of the brain's opiate receptors. The pattern of these receptors, which are concentrated in the spinal cord, the brainstem, and the limbic system of the cerebrum, is found consistently in rats, humans, and other mammals—indeed, throughout the vertebrates. Clearly, a pattern so widely conserved across the evolutionary scale must have value for the animal's survival.

The next question was why the vertebrate brain should come equipped with the ability to "get high" on morphine or heroin. Or, to reframe the question, were the opiates gaining ready access by fitting into receptor sites that were there to serve some other built-in function? If so, the opiates must all be similar in structure—which they are—and they must also resemble the "original" endogenous transmitters well enough to mislead the receptor sites. By this point, armed with a rough sketch of the transmitters' structure and with clues as to their likely function, researchers had a good idea of what they were looking for. In the mid-1970s a handful of natural opiates, collectively termed "endorphins," were identified; they included a group called enkephalins and another group headed by beta-endorphin.

From the perspective of a couple of decades, the endorphin story reads like one of the more straightforward detective novels, in which every clue is found at its proper time and the inquiry moves steadily forward. What was most striking at the time, however, was that the mapping of the receptors, a task that might be thought purely mechanical and unimportant, was what gave this investigation its major impetus. This approach, which uses the mapping of receptor sites as a first step, has proved valuable in other investigations as well, such as studies of the innate function of receptor sites in the brain that bind delta-9 THC (tetrahydrocannabinol), the major psychoactive ingredient in marijuana.

FOCUSING IN ON RECEPTOR SITES

The close study of receptor sites is a lively subfield in itself. Previously unknown techniques of imaging and magnification can go beyond displaying the location of sites in the brain as a whole, down to the molecule-by-molecule layout of a single receptor. And the structures disclosed with these techniques are fascinating. No longer regarded as the passive "lock" of a "lock-and-key" mechanism, the receptors appear to work from a few simple elements and to achieve a wide range of effects.

Robert Lefkowitz and his colleagues at the Howard Hughes Medical Institute at Duke University have been looking closely at epinephrine and norepinephrine receptor sites for several years—practically the lifetime of this field so far. The adrenergic (epinephrine-using) receptors make a good model for studying a more general class of receptors, those that work through the G-proteins and bring about the production of second messengers inside the cell. Adrenergic receptors are found in most mammalian tissues and appear to fall into four types, called alpha-1, alpha-2, beta-1, and beta-2. They are associated with the two second-messenger systems discussed earlier: cyclic AMP and DG–IP$_3$. Specifically, the beta receptors apparently increase the rate of production of cyclic AMP, and the alpha-2 receptors decrease it.

This was roughly the extent of what was known until about 1986. Then Lefkowitz and others succeeded in reading the full genetic sequence of the beta-2 receptor, which allowed them to clone the gene—in effect, to create thousands of copies of the beta-2 receptor in their laboratory.

What they learned in the process was astonishing: a single receptor site spans the cell membrane, like a built-in tunnel, no fewer than seven times. The arrangement consists of seven recurring clusters of 20 to 25 amino acids, each crossing the membrane and all held together by loops of amino acids within the cell and just outside the membrane. This pattern appears to hold good for the other kinds of receptors as well. In a comparison of any two receptors, 40 to 50 percent of the sequence is identical—a high degree of conservation and an indication of how effective this structure must be.

As well as elucidating the fine structure of the beta-2 receptor, the cloning work of Lefkowitz and others turned up at least five more adrenergic receptors, all different from one another (in ways that had been imperceptible before the techniques of molecular genetics) and each with its own functions in the cell. From the point of view of clinical applications, this was, and continues to be, an exciting time for drug research, because it becomes possible to distinguish more closely among receptors and to select medications with increasing specificity. In the future it may even be possible to develop drugs targeted to particular subtypes of receptors and reduce unwanted side effects to a bare minimum.

The arrangement of seven membrane-spanning domains occurs widely throughout nature, in numerous guises. Many hormones, as well as transmitters, have receptors of this type; proteins called the opsins, which are precursors for the visual pigments, also fall in this category; and even in species as distant from ourselves as the slime mold, cyclic AMP is regulated through such a receptor. Meanwhile, with what is already known, many researchers are tackling the question of just what it is about the receptor's structure that determines function.

For questions of this sort, one technique is particularly effective—with the added advantage (or disadvantage, depending on one's taste) of sounding like something from a science fiction script. This technique is the creation of chimeras, creatures or structures that are artificially assembled from diverse genetic origins. Chimeric receptors created with recombinant DNA are excellent tools for study, because they allow the investigator to alter the receptor's structure, one small piece at a time, and then to observe any associated change in functioning. For example, researchers explored the activity of a chimeric receptor made up mostly of the alpha-2 type, with a small portion of beta receptor inserted into it. The receptor bound the substances that would be expected for an alpha receptor, but then it stimulated second-messenger production, as would be expected of a *beta* receptor. Thus, like the original chimera in Greek mythology (part-lion, part-goat, part-serpent),

Neurotransmitter-gated ionic channels

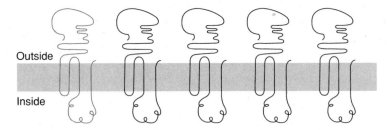

Voltage-gated ionic channels

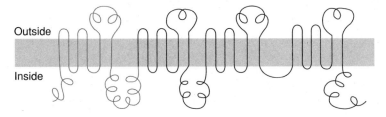

G-protein-coupled receptors

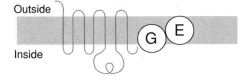

G = G-protein   E = effector protein

FIGURE 5.2.   Receptor sites in the brain exhibit a variety of structures that each correspond with a particular function.   Some (top row) receive the chemical signals of neurotransmitters and convert them into electrical signals, by allowing or halting the flow of charged ions into or out of the cell.   Other receptors (middle) are triggered by electrical signals—changes in voltage—and respond by channeling ions into or out of the cell.   The G-protein-coupled receptors (bottom row) react not to ions or neurotransmitters but to a "second messenger" (the G protein); the result is a chemical reaction that takes place inside the cell and, consequently, a change in the cell's activities.   What all receptor sites apparently have in common is a molecular structure that extends across the cell membrane (gray bar) and back again several times.   The G-protein-coupled receptors span the membrane no fewer than seven times.   Source: Marcus Raichle, Washington University School of Medicine, St. Louis, Mo.

this receptor is a fabrication, a blend of incongruous parts. With continued fine-tuning of the size and precise placement of chimeric insertions, researchers should be able to isolate the specific amino acids in the receptor that determine one or another biological function.

The dynamic nature as well as the versatility of the adrenergic receptors offers appealing avenues for further investigation. For instance, what takes place at the molecular level during the process of desensitization, in which the response drops in intensity over time even though the stimulus remains constant? All the evidence thus far suggests that there may be a new—previously unknown—protein kinase involved in desensitization, which essentially works the "off" switch for a receptor that has bound to a first messenger. Lefkowitz and his coworkers named such a substance, sight unseen, BARK—for beta adrenergic receptor kinase—and then proceeded to find it. BARK cooperated by revealing itself as a distant relative of the second messenger-sensitive protein kinases.

BARK works in cooperation with another newly discovered protein, barrestin (for "beta-arrestin"), to inactivate the receptor site temporarily. The mechanism works in two steps. When BARK is called into action by the binding of a neurotransmitter, it adds a phosphate group to the receptor site, thereby changing its shape. Barrestin can now bind easily to the receptor site and complete the action of the "off" switch.

The proving of a hunch can be its own best reward—particularly for the scientist, who is often pursuing something as intangible as a closer look at some aspect of nature. But the discovery of BARK and barrestin brings a practical bonus. In the development of pharmaceutical aids to reduce desensitization and thereby prolong the therapeutic effect of some drugs, BARK and barrestin offer two targets that were completely unknown only a few years ago.

THE INTRIGUING ROLE OF THE ION CHANNELS

While the discovery of neurotransmitters and elucidation of the structure of their receptor sites have been proceeding apace, another family of receptor sites is also becoming increasingly well known to neuroscience. This family comprises all the voltage-gated channels, so named because they are activated by electricity—voltage differentials across the cell membrane—rather than by chemical factors such as the neurotransmitters. (Some receptors for neurotransmitters are coupled to voltage-gated channels in a sort of duplex arrangement.)

The main voltage-gated channels are of three types: potassium and sodium, by means of which the nerve cell fires an electrical impulse and transmits that impulse along the axon; and calcium, which reacts to the electrical charge at the end of the axon by releasing neurotransmitter into the synaptic cleft. The genetic sequences of these channels are all strikingly similar, even in animals as disparate as mammals and fruit flies. (Fruit flies, in particular, are a boon to the researcher, who can thus tackle many intriguing questions of neurophysiology in an animal model that produces a new generation every two weeks.)

The past few years have seen the emergence of new techniques for studying extremely precise sections of neuroanatomy, such as a particular kind of ion channel, isolated "in the dish," in a laboratory setting. By these means, it may soon be possible to observe what goes on during the process of learning at the cellular level, where nerve cells store information in some physical form for later retrieval. (For an account of recent findings in this field, see Chapter 8.) In addition, a better understanding of the genetic instructions for assembling various ion channels cannot fail to have clinical applications—for example, in the design of drugs for now-irreversible conditions, or in the pinpointing of genetic variations that may predispose an individual toward certain diseases.

Genetic studies have made it possible to clone several ion channels—the optimum method for a close study of channel structure. Cloning of the sodium channel gene has revealed that it includes four domains, each of which spans the membrane multiple times. The calcium channel, too, consistently contains four domains, each with multiple membrane-spanning sequences; the potassium channel shows more variation in form. The protein sequence for the potassium channel also is noticeably smaller, perhaps one-quarter that of the sodium channel.

Experiments in the past few years have shown that the diverse potassium channels tend to share a common core region of their DNA sequence; the differences reside in the terminal regions. Potassium channels with different terminal regions are found in different parts of the brain. Diversity may also arise by another means: several of the relatively short sequences may coalesce in various ways to form a single potassium channel.

The research team of Lily Yeh Jan, at Howard Hughes Medical Institute and the Departments of Physiology and Biochemistry at the University of California, San Francisco, set out to test this possibility. They began by injecting an assortment of genetic material for potassium channels into developing egg cells of *Xenopus*, the African toad. The potassium channels thus created displayed an interesting combination of traits. For example, one set had lost most of the important "inactivation" function: not only did these channels remain open longer than usual but they were liable to open at any time rather than in precise response to a change in electrical polarization of the nerve cell. (Inactivation itself is thought to come about by a sort of molecule-sized tetherball, which swings into the mouth of the open potassium channel and thereby blocks it; negative charges at the mouth of the pore would temporarily hold the particle, which is presumably positively charged, in place. This model is being tested in several laboratories.) Other channels remained open for some time, but only in the first half of the depolarization phase. Clearly, while not all the combinations formed in this way are functional, a great many are. The net result is a great range of possible functions achieved with relative economy of means.

THE CASE OF THE 5-SECOND MESSENGER MOLECULE

In another trail of research, molecular biology and genetics are joining pharmacology to bring to light the workings of yet one more type of messenger molecule. The molecule nitric oxide fills a critical role in diverse tissues of the body, from the lining of blood vessels to the cerebellum, but its identity as a messenger of anything at all was completely unsuspected for a long time. For one thing, the compound—a single atom of nitrogen joined to one atom of oxygen—was very unstable, existing only for a matter of seconds. What could it be doing in the body?

It was the well-known effect of nitroglycerin on intense chest pains that first put investigators on the trail of nitric oxide as a messenger molecule. Nitroglycerin works in remarkably small doses to dilate the blood vessels and relieve chest pain. Pharmacologists already knew that nitric oxide was the active ingredient formed by the body from nitroglycerin. But what became clear only in the late 1980s was that nitric oxide was the very substance being sought independently in cardiovascular research as a "relaxing factor" that works in tandem with the neurotransmitter ACh in the lining of blood vessels. It soon emerged that nitric oxide does not bring about this effect alone; rather it stimulates the production of a second messenger, cyclic GMP (cyclic guanosine monophosphate).

As for its origin, nitric oxide is formed by the action of an enzyme from the amino acid arginine; another acid, citrulline, is given off as a by-product. One of the reasons nitric oxide has been so difficult to find in the body is that it is so short-lived (its half-life is five seconds). But the citrulline that is produced at the same time does remain in the system and it can be measured, providing a clue to the evanescent presence of nitric oxide.

At this point in the inquiry, brain researchers began to take an active interest. Solomon Snyder, director of the neuroscience department at Johns Hopkins Medical School, was intrigued by the actions of nitric oxide, and especially by their extraordinary rapidity. He felt sure a system as remarkable as that of nitric oxide could not have developed only for use in blood vessels—it must also be at work somewhere in the brain.

Snyder's research team used as their starting point the established fact that when the neurotransmitter glutamate binds to receptor sites, the calcium channels open and a great amount of cyclic GMP is produced. Once the investigators knew what to look for, they could follow two lines of evidence simultaneously: levels of citrulline and levels of cyclic GMP, both of which indicate the action of nitric oxide.

Sure enough, stimulating the glutamate receptors in the cerebellum tripled the levels of citrulline and increased the levels of GMP almost tenfold. (Conversely, when the cells were treated with a drug that inhibits the nitric oxide–forming enzyme, no cyclic GMP was produced, even when the glutamate receptors were activated—a check on cause and effect that confirmed the researchers' hunch.) As another piece of evidence, these great increases in cyclic GMP production all took place within a few seconds. This was a remarkably swift reaction, well within the time frame of some of the more brisk neurotransmitters. It appears that the nitric oxide-forming enzyme is switched on as soon as the calcium channels open, and it begins at once to produce nitric oxide at full speed, with some help from calmodulin, a calcium-binding protein.

Thus, nitric oxide is indeed at work in the brain, and it is associated with one of the most important excitatory neurotransmitters—glutamate. Intriguingly, nitric oxide is neither a transmitter nor a second messenger but truly a different type of messenger between cells. By mapping the areas of the brain where the nitric oxide–forming enzyme tends to concentrate, investigators are beginning to understand more about the action of this substance.

Nitric oxide–forming enzyme is found in high concentrations in the cerebellum, which is largely involved in movement, and in the olfactory bulb; it also appears in the pituitary gland (the producer of many hormones), in sections of the eye, and in the intestine (where it may turn out to be the primary agent of muscle relaxation). One of the most exciting of recent results is the finding that certain arteries in the brain contain the enzyme not only in their interior lining but, more unusually, in the neurons that supply the outer layer—the very arteries and nerves recently shown to be involved in migraine headaches. These observations are already being applied in the rapid development of drugs to act at this site in the nitric oxide system, and may soon bring millions of migraine sufferers a new prospect of relief. This novel form of molecular signal, discovered so recently, suggests that there are still more intriguing trails to be explored within the messenger systems.

ACKNOWLEDGMENTS

Chapter 5 is based on presentations by Lily Yeh Jan, Robert Lefkowitz, and Solomon H. Snyder.

6

The Development and Shaping of the Brain

The making of the human brain from the tip of a 3 millimeter neural tube is a marvel of biological engineering. To arrive at the more than 100 billion neurons that are the normal complement of a newborn baby, the brain must grow at the rate of about 250,000 nerve cells per minute, on average, throughout the course of pregnancy. But it is not the volume of growth alone that makes the production of a human brain staggering to consider. The great number of functions that the brain reliably carries out and the specificity with which these are assigned to one or another type of cell or small location in the whole assembly are stunning in their complexity; yet the feat of growing a human brain occurs in hundreds of millions of individuals each year. The brain's 100 trillion or so interconnections provide the physical basis for its speed and sophistication. But how is such an intricate network constructed in the first place? Does the genetic material of the fertilized egg already contain a full set of building specifications for the human brain, in which every cell is created as a minute increment in the overall design? And if the set of instructions is indeed so closed and specific, how could chance or random mutations or the influence of the environment have played a role—as they so evidently have done and continue to do—in the emergence of the *first* human brains?

From these questions, it is easy to see that any scientific account of the development of the human brain has to meet a formidable challenge. For such an account must not only explain a sequence of development of great orderliness and efficacy but also allow room for the creative effects of chance—in the form of random mutations and the ensuing natural selection—that have led to the propagation of this particular form of brain in the first place. The majority of developmental neuroscientists today respond to this challenge by proposing a series of stages in which built-in instructions and the effects of arbitrary external events are mingled to an intriguing degree.

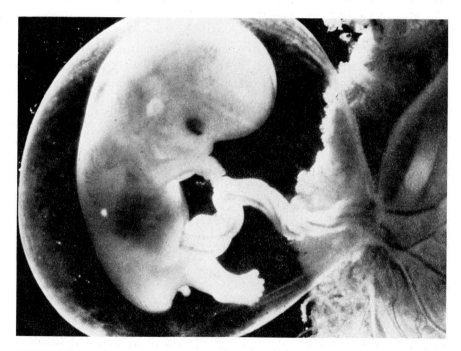

FIGURE 6.1. The development of the human brain during gestation is a highly complex project on a tight schedule. In this 12- to 14-week-old embryo, nerve cells are proliferating at the rate of about 15 million per hour. The physical bases for perception are beginning to emerge: one can make out an eye (the black dot) and the future site of the ear (the white area just above). Source: National Institute of Child Health and Human Development.

According to this scheme, the essential stages are (1) proliferation of a vast number of undifferentiated brain cells; (2) migration of the cells toward a predetermined location in the brain and the beginning of their differentiation into the specific type of cell appropriate to that location; (3) aggregation of similar types of cells into distinct regions; (4) formation of innumerable connections among neurons, both within and across regions; and (5) competition among these connections, which results in the selective elimination of many and the stabilization of the 100 trillion or so that remain. These events do not occur in rigid sequence but overlap in time, from about 5 weeks after conception onward. After about 18 months of age, no more neurons are added, and the aggregation of cell types into distinct regions is roughly complete. But the pruning of excess connections—clearly a process of great importance for the shape of the mature brain—continues for years.

This model of the sequence of brain development has led toward many fruitful lines of investigation in neuroscience. Among other things, it can explain well-known birth defects of the brain or the nervous system in terms of the stage at which development was disturbed. If, for instance, at a very early stage the neural tube fails to close properly, the cells that should form the forebrain and its overlying skull and scalp may not be generated; this condition, anencephaly ("without brain"), almost always results in stillbirth or in survival for only a few hours. Less severe defects of the neural tube may give rise to varying degrees of spina bifida ("split spine"), with the spinal column missing the bony protection of some of its vertebrae. Exposure to x-rays, high levels of alcohol, and some drugs can impair development at crucial early stages, as can the mother's infection with certain diseases such as rubella (German measles).

At about the midpoint of pregnancy, from about 15 to 20 weeks after conception, the number of brain cells in the cerebral cortex increases rapidly; by the seventh month, the fetus is emitting its own brain waves, which can be detected through the mother's abdomen. Several lines of evidence suggest that proper nutrition is of greatest importance for the development of the brain at this stage, although it continues to be crucial until birth and for some time afterward. Yet even when the developing brain suffers environmental insults such as malnutrition, it shows a remarkable capacity to recover and go on to develop normally, provided the harmful circumstances are corrected within the first 3 months or so after birth.

One of the problems facing neuropathologists interested in congenital neurological defects is that they usually examine the brain long after the abnormal events have passed. Another problem is that the "normal" data in this area may cover a wide range of variation. A basic understanding of normal brain development is essential for identifying and addressing those factors that can interfere with the making of a healthy brain.

STUDYING THE BRAIN IN DEVELOPMENT

Short of technology that would shrink a remote video camera down to the size of a cellular implant, how can neuroscientists study brain development as an ongoing process in the living animal? The multistage model is useful here, too, as it was in explaining various brain disorders, because it suggests several points at which researchers can alter the process of development in a highly controlled way and learn a great deal by observing the outcome. Currently, three techniques are working especially well for researchers who want to know more about the making of the cerebral cortex, in particular. One technique is based on the knowledge that all the cells destined to become part of the cerebral cortex are first generated near the center of the brain, at the fluid-filled ventricles that have formed from the original three bulges in the neural tube. If a small number of ventricular cells are removed and labeled with various neutral dyes, then reinjected while cell proliferation is still going on, it is possible to follow a particular group of dyed cells as they migrate to their eventual positions in the cortex. So far, this approach has suggested that a cell may already contain the information of its eventual "address" in the cortex when it is generated; for example, a cell that is removed when the ventricle is producing layer 3 of the cortex and then injected back into the ventricle during the generation of layer 4 will nonetheless migrate to layer 3. Hence, genetic information may strongly control this aspect of development.

A second technique works at the genetic level by inserting

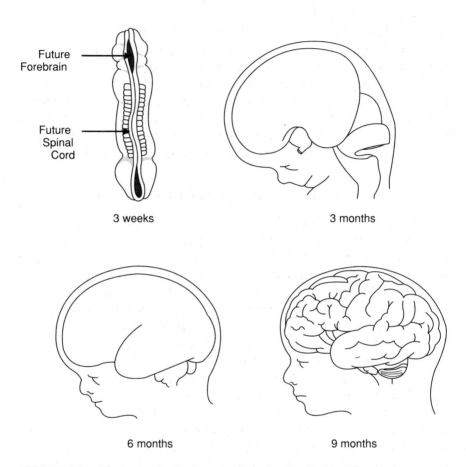

FIGURE 6.2. The human brain develops from the tip of a 3-millimeter-long neural tube. At three to four weeks after conception, the neural groove closes into a tube, and three distinct regions—a hindbrain, midbrain, and forebrain—begin to take form. By three months' gestation, the brain has multiplied in size several times; the forebrain has grown particularly fast and now dwarfs the other regions. At six months, the cerebral cortex overshadows most of the other structures and has begun to separate into lobes. At nine months, with its wrinkled and disproportionately large cortex, the brain is instantly recognizable as human. Underneath the cortex, other specialized structures are also present and in working order.

an innocuous retrovirus into ventricular cells. The retrovirus does not affect normal functioning, but its genetic information is incorporated into the living cells' DNA and faithfully replicated in the cells of future generations. The genetic code of the retrovirus can thus be used as a marker, much as dyes were used in the preceding technique. Here, though, the technique allows an investigator to observe successive generations of cells rather than the spatial distribution of cells that are all from one generation.

The third technique gives dramatic results by knocking out one generation of cells altogether. For example, exposing a pregnant monkey to x-ray irradiation at a particular point in its pregnancy will interfere with cell division at a discrete stage, so that the cells, say, for layer 3 of the limbic cortex are not generated. Subsequent layers are generated and laid down normally, but with a particular population of cells missing in the middle layer, the connections from one part of the brain to another may falter. Thus, the individual may find it difficult to bring together different types of information or to respond appropriately to a stimulus. Disorders of this kind, which have less to do with overall anatomical structure than with the brain's ability to form and use synaptic connections, may play a role in some psychiatric illnesses for which there is no obvious physical cause.

The cerebral cortex is a fascinating object of study from many perspectives. It comprises by far the largest portion of the human brain—about three-quarters, in the adult—and is arguably the single anatomical structure that most sets us apart from other animals, even from other hominoids such as the chimpanzee (with whom we share well over 95 percent of our genetic makeup). Yet apparently no single transmitter or type of cell is unique to the human cerebral cortex; the molecules found in the cortex can also be found elsewhere, in our muscles, heart, and intestines and in the brains of other animals as well. The molecules, and even the cells, may be the same; it is the patterns of connectivity that make a difference. The connections, or synapses, among neurons in the human brain are not only more numerous but also more intricately patterned than anything that has ever been constructed to process information, including the most sophisticated supercomputer.

A structure so complex must be considered in smaller units if it is to be understood at all, and up to now neuroscience has managed to get along quite well with two mutually incompatible systems. One system for subdivision was devised by the German psychiatrist K. Brodmann at the turn of the century. Brodmann distinguished 57 areas of the cortical surface on the basis of their tissue composition, and the reference numbers he assigned are still widely used today. A researcher giving a talk before an international audience of neuroscientists can mention "area 44" and be understood without further explication. The other system subdivides the cortex into areas of specialized function—which do not correspond well to Brodmann's physically discrete areas, unfortunately. Thus, in terms of function, one can refer to Broca's area, which controls the ability to translate thoughts into speech (but not the ability to understand when someone else speaks; that function is housed in Wernicke's area, which is nearby, but not adjacent). The area is defined quite clearly in terms of its function, but its physical extent is harder to outline. In Brodmann's scheme, Broca's area occupies some of area 44 and some of area 45, as well as a little of area 4.

Current techniques of magnification and imaging permit the analysis of different tissues at the molecular level and have added another order of information to an already complicated picture. But this new information may ultimately be the bridge between the functional map of the cerebral cortex and the physical map, because it offers finer distinctions within functional areas and reveals the differential distribution of certain molecules along the lines of function. The molecules being considered are often receptor sites and the particular neurotransmitters that go with them; and (as we have seen in Chapter 5) it is through the neurotransmitters and their receptor sites that the brain translates its countless functions into chemical terms and back again into function. In this regard, the research team of Pasko Rakic at the Yale University School of Medicine has worked extensively with areas 17 and 18, which roughly correspond to the primary visual cortex—the part of the brain that must receive sensory impulses from the eyes before the visual association cortex (located nearby) can tell us what we see or how we feel about it.

In experimenting with differential development, Rakic and

his colleagues have found that neighboring areas can be related in function and yet compete for some of the same resources—namely, territory and energy—so that if chance or environmental circumstances favor it, one area may develop at the expense of another. Clearly, such contests have implications for the shaping of the brain on an evolutionary time scale as well as over the course of an individual's development. Even in the short evolutionary interval from monkeys to humans this kind of reapportionment can be found: for example, the primary visual cortex, which makes up 15 percent of the cerebral cortex in the monkey, accounts for only 3 percent of our own cerebral cortex, while other areas have grown disproportionately larger. Among individuals of the same species, too, and even between the two hemispheres of an individual's brain, there can be variations in the size of a particular area, although nothing like the 3 to 15 percent difference just mentioned. Even when quite subtle, these variations can yield evidence of the intermingled effects on development of genetic information, random mutations, and environmental influences.

MASS PRODUCTION OF BRAIN CELLS

The assembly of a human brain, a complex undertaking on a non-negotiable schedule, calls for a vast number of cells of suitable design, available at a convenient location. Cell proliferation therefore is a critical early stage of brain development, and one in which even small changes—in the timing of a cell-generating cycle, the duration of such a cycle, or the number of cycles altogether—can have major consequences for the final product.

Proliferation takes place largely under the control of regulatory genes, which act primarily to affect the operation of other, structure-building genes. The first structures laid down contain some of the specifications for the more advanced structures of the next stage, and so on. In this way, the genetic coding that sets a developmental process in motion need not contain *all* the information expressed in the final structure—only enough to move the process along to a point where a fresh element (such as a hormone or a neurotransmitter newly accessible to the developing structure) can provide further specifications.

Brain cells proliferate according to a scheme that combines order with enormous productivity. In the ventricular zone, a small number of precursor cells divide in two; then, in another cycle, each precursor cell divides again, perhaps several more times. The effect of each cycle at this stage is to double the number of cells; therefore, adding even a single cycle, for example by extending the duration of this early proliferative stage, could make a great difference in the overall size of the brain. As it happens, the difference in size between a monkey's cerebral cortex and that of a human can be accounted for by just a little more than three such cycles. And indeed, the entire neuron-generating stage, including these early cycles that immediately double the number of cells as well as later cycles in which multiplication proceeds more slowly, does seem to follow this rationale in its timing. The neuron-generating process in both monkeys and humans begins on about the 40th day after conception; the process ceases in monkeys on about the 100th day but continues in humans for about another 25 days.

By contrast, adding an extra few cycles at a later stage would have a much less striking effect, because by then most cells are dividing asymmetrically; that is, each cell produces one daughter (which does not divide) and one progenitor (which does). Furthermore, by the late stages, most of the cells have migrated to their eventual positions and are aggregating into the cerebral cortex. An extra couple of cell divisions at this point would produce not more surface area, which is the essential property of a larger cortex, but only an extra layer of cells on top of the surface that is already taking shape.

One of the reasons for this limitation, and a guiding principle in the construction of the brain, is that the proliferative ventricular zone apparently holds information about both the quantities of various cells needed and their eventual function or location. Pasko Rakic and his colleagues propose that somewhere in the mosaic of the ventricular zone is a protomap of the future regions of the brain, including the cerebral cortex. This map is actually better understood as a series of columns packed closely together on the surface of the cerebral ventricles. The precursor cells divide in two while at the ventricular surface and then move off to synthesize a full complement of DNA; afterward, they shuttle back to the surface to undergo another cell division. This process is repeated numerous times, until about the 100th day of gestation of a rhesus monkey, for example. But the end of cell proliferation does not mean that the columns have outlived their usefulness. On the contrary, they are essential for the accuracy of the next, and in some ways most remarkable, stage in the development of the cerebral cortex.

MIGRATION TO THE CEREBRAL CORTEX

The mammalian brain develops from the core outward. Long before the recognizably wrinkled surface of the cerebral cortex appears, the hollow, fluid-filled ventricles are present. These serve both as a connection back to the spinal cord (and a reminder of the still earlier neural tube) and as the site of origin for the new elements that will ultimately be assembled into the outermost surface of the brain, the cerebral cortex. Thus, in the course of development, the neurons and supporting glial cells of the cortex must somehow make their way there from the ventricular zone. This stage has been described as a massive migration of cells, and the distances involved are enormous, at least from the point of view of a single cell: some may travel as much as several millimeters to their eventual destination in the cortex.

But how does the cell "know" its eventual destination? Pasko Rakic suggests that the columns play an important role here. More specifically, the columns that make up the protomap at the ventricular surface could be seen as including a proliferative unit at the base and then a cellular pathway along which nerve cells travel when they have stopped dividing and begun to mature. As the neurons of each unit migrate along the pathway in a set order and settle into position in the cortex, they would reproduce faithfully the orderly arrangement of the units in which they originated—a feature termed cytoarchitectonic, for "architecture of the cells." According to this model, the surface area (even if convoluted) of each region of the cerebral cortex would be a function of the number of proliferative units contributing to it, whereas the thickness of the cortex at any particular spot would depend on the number of cell-division cycles that occurred within a unit. As an example, the primary visual cortex of the monkey comprises roughly 2.5 million such units, each containing about 100 to 120 cells. (These are arranged in the characteristic six layers of the cerebral cortex described in Chapter 2.)

A migrating neuron is guided along its set pathway by special adhesion molecules arrayed on a temporary framework of supporting (glial) cells. The glial cells composing the pathways for most neurons are extremely elongated and stringy in form, making a dense radial pattern from the ventricular zone to the outer layers of the developing brain. Once the stage of migration is accomplished, some of these glial cells degenerate; others undergo cell division and join the mature network of supporting cells, the "white matter," in the brain. Although occasionally a migrating neuron may transfer from one set of radial glial fibers to another en route, most of the time the adhesion molecules are strong enough to keep a neuron in the path to which it first became attached from the ventricular zone and to draw the neuron without entanglement through the dense arrangement of other cells, axons, and dendrites that are accumulating in the cortex.

A smaller number of cells are apparently uninfluenced by the radial glial pathways and instead follow a different set of paths by adhering to the surface of axons. These cells are likely to migrate along the outer margin of the brain, perpendicular to the radial glial pathways; they may migrate from one region to another or even across the midline that divides the two hemispheres. Clearly, a different set of adhesion molecules is responsible for this type of migration, which helps to form several important elements of the pons and the medulla in the brainstem, for example. Even more unusual is the sort of migration by which the cerebellum is formed: the granule cells that form a layer in the "little brain" at the back of the head show affinities for both axonal and glial surfaces and, in effect, combine the two forms of migration. The exceptional approach of the granule cell makes it a good case study for the mechanics and other properties at work in preferential cell adhesion.

One other striking aspect of neuronal migration is the order in which the six layers of the cortex are built up: from the innermost to the outermost. Each migrating neuron, before arriving at its own predetermined site in the cortex, must travel outward through all the neurons that have migrated and settled in the cortex before it. As a result, each layer of the cortex, as it builds up, has the opportunity to carry an accretion of information from nearby cells that have preceded it— information that may help to lay the groundwork for the next developmental stage.

THE FORMATION OF SYNAPSES AND REGIONS

After migration, the tendency of recently arrived neurons to cluster with similar cells into distinct regions determines the form and ultimately the function of each part of the brain. At the upper and outer surface, the cortical sheet becomes continuous at this stage and begins to compress into its characteristic folds and creases, as more cells from the proliferative units continue to add surface area to an already crowded space. The various types of cells also finish differentiating, so that each type has the biochemical properties, receptor sites, and other features appropriate to its region and layer. The cell body of the neuron grows longer and extends its axon (for transmitting signals to a target cell) and it also puts forth numerous branching dendrites (for receiving signals and conveying them back to the cell body).

The process of aggregation is highly ordered. Cells of the same type recognize one another and draw together; in many populations of neurons, cells may even arrange themselves with the same orientation. (For example, the large pyramidal neurons in the cerebral cortex that transmit impulses to other regions tend to align themselves with their axons extended toward the underlying white matter and their dendrites pointing toward the surface.) Additionally, in at least some contexts, axons tend to grow in bundles, or "fasciculations," closely associated with one another; they dissociate somewhat as they approach their target neurons, which suggests that there may be some form of recognition molecules, and possibly adhesion molecules as well, along the surface of axons.

Most important, the cells form synapses or connections with one another. As discussed in Chapter 2, a synapse may occur between the axon of one neuron and the dendrite of another, between the axon of one neuron and the cell body of another, or between axons or dendrites themselves. Synapses also form between cell bodies directly, for the exchange of signals by electrical impulse rather than through neurotransmitters (see Chapter 2). Whatever the nature of the synapses, it is their universality—the degree to which they connect everything with everything—that makes the human brain such a superb integrator of information. The burgeoning of synapses in all directions is at least partly directed by several messenger molecules, which are also to be found in the adult nervous system. In the mature brain they may act, for example, as second messengers broadcasting a signal within the cell, or as neuromodulators influencing the way a signal is received at a synapse. But at the aggregation stage of the developing brain, these compounds have other effects, such as enhancing the site recognition that may precede the forming of a synapse, or supplying nutrition to the nerve cell as it is forming a synapse.

The target cell toward which an axon is growing can also help with synapse formation by providing some of the chemical compounds needed by the axon. The best-known of these compounds is nerve growth factor, which the axon takes up by means of specific receptors and transports back to its cell body. A cell nourished with nerve growth factor may have an advantage at the next stage of development, when large numbers of cells will be eliminated. Conversely, cells sensitive to nerve growth factor tend to retract their axons from target cells that do not supply it.

Outside the nervous system, other factors contribute to the development of the brain by their influence on the forming of synaptic connections. The fetus itself, in kicking, turning, and (by the fifth month) even sucking its thumb, stimulates the growth of synapses. In addition, at this stage, some conditions of the environment can act directly on the fetal senses: temperature, pressure, and even a rudimentary kind of hearing (although the auditory association cortex is not yet equipped to make sense of what the fetus "hears").

CELLULAR COMPETITION

Taken together, all these growth-enhancing factors (and perhaps others that are not yet identified) give rise to an overproduction of neurons, as well as of everything associated with them: axons, dendrites, the signal-receiving spines on dendrites, and every form of synapse. For example, the developing brain of the rhesus monkey, midway through gestation, has more than twice as many axons as the brain of an adult monkey. In our own species, it is estimated that the newborn arrives with trillions of synapses in her teeming head, a great many of which will cease to exist over the next 12 years or so. Yet far from indicating a loss of function or a decline in brainpower in childhood, the long-drawn-out process of selection is the final essential stage in the development of a nervous system unique to each individual. This uniqueness is a physical fact: the full universe of synaptic connections that takes form in any given human brain reflects the sum of the influences—genetic, nutritional, toxic, environmental, social, psychological, educational, and even accidental—that have all converged, unpredictably and irreproducibly, during the development of this particular brain. The elimination of great numbers of synapses, along with some neurons themselves, is a process widely observed among mammals (and among some other vertebrates as well); thus it appears that the large quantity of synapses present in the brain at birth does not represent the optimum number for a lifetime but rather serves the purpose of providing some room for selection.

This is not to say, however, that some populations of cells and synapses are somehow destined to remain and become permanent while others are programmed to exist only briefly. Instead, in an enactment of Darwinian natural selection at the cellular level, synapses and even neurons compete for survival.

Once we recognize that the early quantities of neurons and synapses are larger than optimal, the outlines of such a competition are easier to see. The population is overly large (in humans, the period of excess synapses continues until about 18 months of age); the territory cannot be expanded (the skull poses definite boundaries); and therefore, individuals must compete for limited resources.

The resources at issue are probably relatively few: nourishment from the target cell (such as nerve growth factor, discussed above), available space on the membrane surface of a target cell, and nerve impulses themselves, which convey information back to the targeting cell body and thereby stimulate its growth. The type of resource that would be crucial for a given synapse depends, of course, on which type of synapse it is. The contest goes on at all levels: a single neuron may first establish communication with its target cell by means of several axons, only one of which will ultimately survive; or a single dendrite may initially receive signals from a neighboring neuron on many dendritic spines, some of which will be eliminated with the onset of maturity. Axons may be retracted (as mentioned earlier), broken down, and absorbed back into the cell for reuse. Alternatively, axons or dendrites, or even whole cell bodies, may simply be allowed to die (most likely from a lack of nourishing factors, rather than of space or stimulation). Eventually they are cleared from the system like other cellular debris.

The cells thus eliminated may include not only those that have lost out in the competition for resources but also some that have misread directional cues at the time of migration and have made their way into inappropriate settings. Some ectopias, as these abnormally situated cells are called, remain in place and can contribute to several recognizable disorders of brain development; most are eliminated. The stage of selective cell death thus provides an opportunity to correct errors as well as a means of sculpting a nervous system into its unique shape.

Although such sculpting may achieve quite precise ends as it eliminates excess cells and synapses, it also goes well beyond the level of slight adjustments here and there. The extent of this process is difficult to comprehend in the abstract. To reduce it to more concrete terms, the Rakic research group has looked at the rate of destruction specifically in the corpus callosum, the tough bundle of nerve fibers that connects the two hemispheres of the brain. In the adult macaque monkey, this bundle contains about 50 million axons. But the macaque brain at birth contains about 200 million axons in this same area. To reach the level at which it functions in adulthood, the corpus callosum apparently eliminates axons at a very high rate—about 60 per second in infancy, for example. Synapses are lost at a much higher rate, since each branching axon could form several points of contact with a target cell. For the human brain, each of these numbers should probably be multiplied by about 10; but the principle of competitive elimination is the same.

The stage of elimination is extensive in another way, too, affecting not only synapses, axons, dendrites, or whole neurons but also receptor sites for specific neurotransmitters—again, an effective way of regulating the functions of the cell. Pasko Rakic and his co-workers plotted development in three regions of the cerebral cortex—motor, visual, and association—in the monkey and found that the number of receptors for dopamine first rose sharply and then fell, in parallel with the synapses and cells and also in parallel with the levels of dopamine itself in the region. Clearly, this stage of widespread destruction—which involves great waste and yet is essential for proper functioning—still presents some puzzles for investigators.

EXPLORING NEW AREAS

The sequence of development in the human brain is much better understood than it was even 20 years ago. Suitably, as the several developmental stages themselves have been found to overlap considerably in their timing, researchers are pursuing investigations into several aspects of the process simultaneously. In the Rakic laboratory, along with work on migration, aggregation, and the end-stage shaping of the nervous system, researchers are also inquiring into a very early stage. How are cells of, for example, the cortical plate (which will ultimately develop into the cerebral cortex) directed to differentiate into one of the six distinct cell types of the cortex and to migrate to the particular layer inhabited by that cell type? There are many hypotheses as to how this specificity comes about. One possible explanation is that all the cells of the cortical plate are equal and undifferentiated until axons from other areas of the brain form synapses with them, thereby leading them to develop into the appropriate target cells. An explanation almost the opposite of this has the development of a cell being prescribed, down to the last detail, in its genetic make-up. Between these two extremes is the possibility that genetic instructions and other developmental events *each* have some part in specifying the form and fate of a cell.

Tests to establish the roles of such tangled factors in brain development pose special problems because of the many orders of information present in highly condensed form. An experimental lesion in one area might effectively isolate the region to be studied, but it could also affect nearby or connected areas, adding unknown factors to the situation under study. Rakic's team, however, found that removing part or all of the optic nerve during development yields a predictable and precise result: the part of the thalamus that relays nerve impulses from the retina to the primary visual cortex grows to be smaller than usual, as does the specific part of the cortex to which it projects (area 17, according to Brodmann's scheme). In the cortical plate, however, everything develops as usual, and the border between areas 17 and 18 also appears to be intact; the number of cells per proliferative unit is its usual 120 or so. Yet although the overall territory of areas 17 and 18 shows no change, the two areas are no longer equal in size, as they would be under normal circumstances; instead, area 17 is proportionately smaller.

There are several ways to account for this. In the absence of live signals to area 17, cells that were originally set to become part of that area may have shifted their development to become part of area 18 instead. In this case, not only would area 18 be larger than the damaged area 17, it would also be larger than the *normal* area 18. However, what the investigators actually found was a smaller-than-usual area 17, a normal-sized area 18—and a new area that was neither one nor the other. This "area x" is distinct from both its neighbors in many respects, including the number of cells in some of its six layers; nevertheless it appears to be something of a hybrid.

Significantly, the synaptic connections formed between area x and any other region of the brain are, by definition, novel. This statement, bland though it may sound, actually holds exciting possibilities—for it offers an explanation of how entirely new cortical regions could have formed during the course of evolution. New cortical areas can be created by a mutation that controls cell proliferation when radial units are being formed. Such areas have the chance for specialization, and whole new sets of synapses transmitting information to and from these areas could prove advantageous now and again; and, if inheritable, they could spread through a population. In this way, the cortical map offering the greatest number of areas that are of use to a particular species would move to become the norm for that species. Although such a model for the emergence of the human brain does not lend itself to replication in the laboratory, it can indeed be tested—for example, by comparing it with evidence from paleoanthropological fossils or by computer simulations. Within the span of an individual lifetime, too, the novel connections of an area x can have implications for the unique circuitry of one person's brain. For example, the cortex of someone who is congenitally blind might include a less-developed area 17 and, perhaps within it or nearby, a hybrid area with novel connections and the possibility of novel functioning.

In neuroscience, study of the formation and development of the human brain holds a special place; many lines of investigation converge here. New methods in molecular biology may now make it possible to uncover specialized genes, for example, that may control cell production in the ventricular zone or regulate the deployment of cell adhesion or cell recognition molecules along migratory pathways. Another set of genes under investigation may initiate the synthesis of neurotransmitters, receptors, and second messengers, and fix the timing for their emergence. Scientists are working, too, on the genes responsible for programmed cell death.

The study of brain development poses its own constraints and appears at times to offer only the most tentative conclusions because of the large number of variables that may all be operating at once. Nevertheless, it also offers a unique vantage point from which to observe the interaction of these same variables—from nutrition all the way down to genetic coding—in their countless possible combinations. At the same time, through its multistage model, this field of inquiry seeks to explain well-known disorders of the brain or nervous system in terms of disturbances at particular points in development. Developmental neuroscience thus forms connections with all its neighboring areas and beyond, much like the system it is observing. No wonder that some of the researchers who specialize in this area think that learning about how the human brain takes shape is "the ultimate study of mankind."

ACKNOWLEDGMENT

Chapter 6 is based on presentations by Pasko Rakic.

7

From Perception to Attention

Although a fair amount is now known about the densely interconnected systems of information processing that reside inside our heads, the coordinated approach of neuroscience still represents a new arrival on the research front. According to David Hubel, professor of neurobiology at Harvard Medical School, the present state of knowledge about some parts of the brain is like that of a visitor from, say, another civilization who sets out to understand everything there is to know about a television set. Such a person may have learned all about transmitters, capacitors, conductors, and properties of resistance—but he is still at a loss, because not only is he unaware of large areas of the circuitry, he still does not know what the television set as a whole is used for. In like manner, basic research on the brain has provided an understanding of how signals are transmitted at the cellular level and identified several types of synapses, as well as an increasing number of neurotransmitters. Yet at a higher level of complexity, much is still unknown about the functions of the central nervous system.

The systems of perception—vision, hearing, taste, smell, and touch—stand as a piquant challenge to researchers in this regard, because they each start from such a well-defined physical basis but then follow exceedingly intricate pathways, bringing in new forms of information at each step, and arriving finally in the realm of subjective experience. Thus the workings of the senses pass at some point beyond the reach of the experimental scientist, because the results can never be reproduced exactly; once information from the brain's association cortex is brought in, the body is no longer simply taking part in some reaction predictable from the laws of physics. Rather, the mind is perceiving something, and the perception is uniquely shaped by that perceiving mind, at that moment.

Nevertheless, scientific research can do a great deal to unravel the pathways of perception, clarifying how and along what lines the information is organized. Vision, the best understood of the perceptive systems, can be explained with confidence well beyond the action of light on the rods and cones of the retina. And some of the mechanisms of this system turn out to be active in other aspects of our conscious behavior as well—namely, in spatial perception and the specific state of mind known as attention.

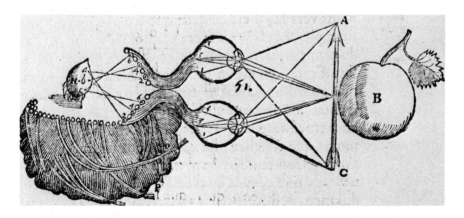

FIGURE 7.1. Explaining the workings of our five senses is a challenge that has been taken up from time to time by natural historians or philosophers. For example, in the seventeenth century, Réné Descartes hypothesized that we are able to see because the nerves project an object from the eyes into the brain, where it is perceived by the soul. Source: Réné Descartes, 1664. *Un Traitté de la Formation du Foetus du Mesme Autheur*. The National Library of Medicine.

PATHWAYS OF INFORMATION IN THE VISUAL SYSTEM

Within the visual system, researchers seek to explain our seamless perception of a three-dimensional surround that contains color, movement, and shape, all assembled from the action of light on our two eyes. What takes place in the rest of the brain, beyond the 125 million rods and cones of each retina, to transmit nerve impulses and organize them into useful messages, recognizable forms, and meaningful scenes?

A basic organizing principle of the visual system is that of a hierarchy of information: a relatively large number of specialized cells at each stage supply information to a smaller number of cells at the next stage, which in turn have their own specialized function. The retinal rods are most attuned to dim light, the cones to bright light (or color). Both rods and cones transmit impulses to another layer of the retina, which sends signals through the third layer to the many neuronal fibers that make up the optic nerve.

Each cell in the third layer that supplies the optic nerve already represents the confluence of signals from thousands of rods and cones over about 1 square millimeter of the retina. The square millimeter thus covered is called the receptive field of that cell. The optic nerve in turn supplies a large amount of pooled information to the lateral geniculate nucleus, which then relays signals to the primary visual cortex.

It is in the primary visual cortex, located in the occipital lobes at the back of the head, that the brain first begins to assemble something that looks like an image to our conscious awareness. At the same time, this area of the cerebral cortex sends many signals to neighboring areas, each of which projects to several others. Without this set of lateral associations, in addition to the hierarchical arrangement, we would not be able to name what we see, for example, or to know whether we had ever seen it before.

This pathway of information, from light beam to nerve impulse to vision, extends for several centimeters inside the human skull and is traversed in thousandths of a second. Along the way, it passes through eight to ten branching stages that consolidate information from the preceding layer into the next one. At the optic chiasm, it branches in another way: half the nerve fibers from each retina cross the brain's midline and lead to the visual cortex of the other hemisphere. The result is that information from the right visual field (gathered by the left half of each eye) is projected to the left visual cortex, and information from the left visual field (the right half of each retina) is projected to the right visual cortex. This arrangement may at first seem overly elaborate, but in fact it offers two advantages. Each half of the brain is responsible for vision on the same side of the body as the hand, arm, and leg for which it controls motor functions; and since each eye provides some signals for the visual cortex in each hemisphere, blindness in one eye, although a serious deprivation, does not mean the loss of the entire left or right visual field.

A curious fact, as yet unexplained, is that at many of these branching stages, a small number of cells project their axons backward, to the preceding stage. The function of this back projection, which allows cells to transmit signals back to the layer from which they came, has puzzled researchers for some time. Could this be some sort of cellular mechanism for checking the "accuracy" of signals as each stage feeds into the next? At present, there are no major hypotheses directing investigations of the matter. But in the other direction—the main flow of signals from the retina to the visual cortex—scientific understanding has improved steadily over the past few decades.

It is quite clear, for example, that the retinal ganglion cells, whose axons are the fibers that make up the optic nerve, sit at a crucial junction in the pathway of information. The retinal ganglion cells act as gatekeepers: their inhibition or excitation determines which signals are sent through the optic nerve, toward the cortex.

The patterns of responsiveness among retinal ganglion cells can vary strikingly, depending on which aspect of vision is being handled. One major pattern is that of center and surrounding area: the retinal cell is stimulated when a small central portion of its receptive field receives light but is inhibited from sending signals when all the area surrounding the center receives light. The reverse may also be true: the center of the receptive field may be inhibited by light, and the surrounding area stimulated by it. Either way, the center-surround pattern responds to *contrast*; the ganglion cell measures not how much light, in absolute terms, is striking the receptive field but how great the difference is between the light in the center and that in the surround. An average amount of light spread out evenly over the whole receptive field thus conveys very little information to this type of cell, which by its nature is much better suited to register detail and the edges of objects.

Another major pattern is instrumental in explaining color vision. Some retinal ganglion cells receive their signals from a mixture of cones, a portion of which are sensitive to light of long wavelengths (that is, red), while others are more sensitive to short wavelengths (blue and green). If the synapses from the long-wavelength cones are excitatory and those from the short-wavelength cones are inhibitory, the result for a ganglion cell would be that reds excite it, blues and greens inhibit it, and white light (which contains a mixture of all the wavelengths) leaves it largely unaffected. This pathway is clearly specialized for one type of information—color—as distinct from the pathway described in the paragraph above, which could be called sensitive to "shape" or "outline."

But the pathway of information for "shape" is not all that straightforward. It includes two subsystems, which correspond to two distinct types of cell in the lateral geniculate (the relay center from the optic nerve to the visual cortex). In each square millimeter of the cortex itself are approximately 100,000 cells—some 80 percent of which do not work by the center-surround design but instead respond best to lines. Contrast is still important: dark lines on a light background, or light lines on a dark background, are the most easily perceived. But another element enters the picture: the *orientation* of the line, whether it is vertical, horizontal, or any number of degrees in between. Small groups of cells each respond best to their own favored orientation, which is mapped in great detail in the cortex: every 50 microns (millionths of a meter) or so, the orientation favored by the cells rotates through about 10 degrees. (In everyday terms, 10 degrees of rotation is equal to one-third the distance between the "1" and "2" on a clock face.) Thus a full 360-degree rotation is described within each half-millimeter or so of the visual cortex.

SEEING THE PATTERNS IN VISUAL SIGNALS

How does the brain coordinate such a flood of information from the eyes? This is a job for the cortex—specifically, the intermediate layers of the primary visual cortex. (The cortex is made up of six layers of cells, as described in Chapter 2; those of most interest here are layers 2 and 4, the neuron-rich granular layers that make synaptic connections within the same localized region.) Signals from the optic nerve pass through the lateral geniculate to the intermediate layers of the cortex, where any given cell receives impulses from either the right or the left eye. Small groups of cells responsive to one eye or the other form a striped pattern in the cortex, which can be made visible by injecting one eye of an anesthetized animal with a radioactive amino acid, exposing it to light, and developing the emitted radiation as a photographic image. The stripes, like the cell groups that respond to a particular orientation of line, are about half a millimeter in diameter.

In the context of right-eye or left-eye responsiveness, the stripes in the cortex are known as ocular dominance columns—indicating a preference toward receiving signals from one eye or the other but not an absolute predetermination. In fact there is some flexibility in the development of this system, especially in the first few years of life. This "plasticity," as it is known in developmental terms, derives in part from the competition among excess numbers of synapses, dendrites, axons, and whole nerve cells described in Chapter 6. The net result for the visual system is that one eye may develop its circuitry more extensively than the other if it has received more stimulation during the crucial early period. David Hubel and his colleagues at the Harvard Medical School demonstrated this phenomenon in an experimental animal by suturing closed one of its eyes shortly after birth. When they opened the eye after several months and injected it with a radioactive substance, the stripes of cortex receiving signals from that eye appeared significantly narrower than normal; the stripes from the other eye were correspondingly wider.

The implications of this work have led to an important change in the treatment of babies born with strabismus (walleye or cross-eye). In such cases, the brain has difficulty coordinating information from the two eyes, and consequently the circuitry of one eye may compete ineffectively for synapses and cells in the visual cortex—even to the point of blindness through underdevelopment of its neural circuitry. In fact, strabismus is a common cause of childhood blindness in the United States. Treatment to prevent this—eye exercises, an eye patch, or corrective surgery to bring the eyes into alignment—is no longer delayed until the age of four, as had been traditional, but now takes place as early as possible, while the neural circuitry underlying vision is still developing.

The systems for ocular dominance and for preferred orientation are of course only two of the patterns of information processing that make up the visual system as a whole. Also embedded in the same portion of the cerebral cortex are systems for color vision, discussed briefly above, and for the perception of depth and movement. Moreover, as will be evident shortly, our sense of ourselves as three-dimensional beings and our orientation in space depend on nerve cells of the visual system. The compactness of information in this system is a marvel of biological engineering, and it overwhelms standard approaches to the investigation of physiology—even those that are extremely precise and that focus on highly localized functions. David Hubel, for example, feels that researchers eventually will need to observe the workings of single nerve cells and to identify the functions of each one, if neuroscience is ever to give a full account of any of the human sensory systems. The level of resolution required for such observations would be much higher than anything available today from the best PET scans or nuclear magnetic resonance imaging. For this area of research, the questions are already at least partly evident, and the technology is racing to catch up.

As mentioned earlier, the brain's system for vision is probably the best understood of the five sensory systems. The pathway of information can be traced from the external stimulus through the sensory organs and along the neural circuitry all the way to conscious perception, and most of the major steps can be sketched in at least lightly. Some features that have first been described for vision will probably be found in other systems as well; for instance, columns or stripes, similar to those of ocular dominance or of line orientation, clearly figure in other systems of the brain (as just one example, see Goldman-Rakic's account of cognition in Chapter 8). But the visual system also has unique properties—the occipital lobe, in which it is mainly located, even looks different from other tissues of the brain—and it continues to engage researchers in its own right. David Hubel, Margaret Livingstone, and their colleagues at Harvard Medical School are exploring the intricacies of an area of the visual cortex that adjoins the one on which they have worked for many years. What circuitry does it have in common with its neighbor? Why is it a distinct area—what does it do differently? Much remains to be discovered in the field of vision research.

THE BRAIN'S SYSTEM FOR SPATIAL PERCEPTION

In addition to the neural circuitry that serves the five primary senses, the human brain has numerous other systems for making sense of external stimuli and regulating the body's ability to function in the world. Although they may produce no obvious perceptions, as does vision or the sense of smell, such systems are often highly sophisticated, drawing on several specialized areas of the brain. An example is the system for visual spatial perception, which most of us take for granted when it is working well. We walk or run, put out a hand to greet an approaching friend, even drive a car along a highway—all the while monitoring the spatial surround. No matter how much or how fast we change our position, we continue to perceive ourselves as being at the center of a space, and to gauge accordingly our spatial relations to other people and to objects in the surround. A measure of the system's sophistication is that this ongoing computation hardly ever requires conscious effort; only when illness or injury interferes with it may we become aware of this vital faculty.

As another measure of sophistication, the system integrates signals from the individual's own body structure and muscle groups, as well as from the sense of sight. The signals from these various sources do not all carry equal weight, however, as was learned from work done in the 1970s by A. Berthoz and his colleagues in Paris and by J. Lishman and D. Lee in Edinburgh. The experiment was simple: subjects walked on a treadmill while scenery was projected on the walls, in the field of their peripheral vision, as if it were moving forward faster than they were walking. Although the subjects' legs were indeed carrying them forward on the treadmill, they reported the sensation of walking *backward*. It seems that visual input overpowered the other signals, although the sensation from the muscle groups involved in walking did contribute to the brain's account of what was going on.

An experimental setting of this kind, in which different forms of information are deliberately set at odds, offers researchers a valuable glimpse of how the brain ordinarily coordinates them. Outside the laboratory, disorders of the spatial perception system take many forms; often they occur without any evident defect in vision or movement. They may appear to be disorders of attention or of "neglect," in a specialized medical sense: the patient ignores or disowns part of her own body, even going so far as to say something like, "Doctor, who put this arm in bed with me?" Striking as such behavior is, the body's ability to recover normal function is equally impressive; in many cases, the patient recovers near-normal functioning within a year.

The cause of such difficulties in the first place is usually an injury to the parietal lobe of the brain, the site of a variety of functions. In one hemisphere (usually, but not always, the left), the parietal lobe controls language. The other hemisphere is associated with such functions as the recognition of shapes and textures and other visual information that is hard to put into words; it also monitors the opposite side of the body and the external environment. A large assortment of disorders, from the severe case described above to more benign (though still distressing) forms, such as the inability to pour a liquid accurately into a glass, have traditionally been collected under the term "parietal lobe syndrome." But a more current view, held, for example, by Vernon Mountcastle and his research team at the Johns Hopkins Medical School, is that this is not a disorder of one discrete lobe of the brain but of a system. Mountcastle, who studies the brain's means of spatial perception, has gathered evidence from numerous research projects that the parietal lobe forms part of a complex distributed system by which the brain actually "constructs" reality. A person stores information about his or her own material dimensions and the three-dimensional surround in several regions of the brain, but the parietal lobe figures importantly in gaining access to that information and in bringing it together effectively.

That the parietal lobe is a major element in this system was demonstrated in another ingenious experiment, this time in the Milan laboratory of E. Bisiach. Here native Milanese citizens were presented with a thought experiment in which they were to imagine themselves standing in the Piazza del Duomo in Milan facing its venerable cathedral, the Duomo. When shown an overview of the buildings around the square, subjects with an injury of the right parietal lobe could not identify the buildings on the left side of the square—that part of their field of vision corresponding to the site of their injury—although these buildings had been familiar to them for years. But when Bisiach asked these subjects to imagine themselves on the *opposite* side of the square, so that right and left were reversed, they could now name the buildings they had previously not been able to identify—and they were unable to name those they had known before. An information system of such fluidity and sensitivity to differing conditions argues for complex circuitry between the parietal lobe and other areas of the brain. In fact, extraordinarily dense connections have been found between two areas of the parietal lobe and parts of the frontal lobe involved in mental representations, planning, and cognition (see Chapter 8).

MAKING SENSE OF MOVEMENT

Studying this kind of perception is a subtle endeavor for the researcher, because although visual stimuli are involved, the point of interest is not the visual system itself but something more like peripheral vision, or spatial awareness. To investigate the "visual neurons of the parietal lobe," Vernon Mountcastle has worked with primates, whose brain structure and sense of sight are much like our own. One experimental approach is to seat the monkey in front of a screen, with an interesting sight projected in the center of the screen to fix the animal's attention. Meanwhile, lights or other displays are moved around in the monkey's peripheral vision to test for particular responses of the visual neurons in the parietal lobe. For more direct observations, it is possible to implant several microelectrodes in the parietal cortex so that each records the activity of a single nerve cell. (The two approaches complement each other because these precise, single-cell recordings are even more informative when examined in the context of observed behavior.)

With this combined approach, Mountcastle has identified several distinct classes of cells in the parietal lobe. One class is active when the animal fixes its attention on a visual target, although these cells do not respond indiscriminately to visual stimuli per se; another class is active when the animal "tracks" a moving target with its eyes; and the third class responds to visual stimuli as such. The neural circuitry between the visual system and the parietal lobe is quite complex and clearly indicates two-way exchange, rather than one area simply feeding into another. Visual neurons of the parietal lobe have their own unique properties: they are highly sensitive to motion, shifts in attention, and the angle of gaze. Unlike neurons of the visual system proper, however, they are rather insensitive to such details as the color, size, or orientation of a visual stimulus.

Electrical recordings from single cells have enabled Mountcastle and his colleagues to work out the pattern by which parietal visual neurons are organized—a pattern quite different from that of the visual cortex itself. In the parietal lobe, a visual neuron will respond, within its receptive field, to a light moving in any of several directions—depending on whether the light is moving toward or away from the center of the field. The center itself apparently is inhibitory for such a cell, giving an overall pattern that, in Mountcastle's words, resembles the outline of a volcano. As a light moves toward the center, the nerve cell increases its response, climbing a slope of excitation—until the light reaches the center and the cell's response drops steeply. Then, as the light continues to move and leaves the center behind, the cell's response starts at a high point again and descends a slope on the other side of the central pit.

This pattern of response appears to take account of the direction of motion in a very idiosyncratic way—it simply registers whether a stimulus is moving toward or away from the center of a particular cell's receptive field. How could such an arrangement possibly give rise to a general perception of the direction in which a visual stimulus is moving? Mountcastle proposes that an accurate signal can be derived even from these imprecise elements, through a simple summing up of the linear vectors. Although there is no way to test this model directly in experimental animals, it has been tested in computer simulations, so far with encouraging results. It appears likely that some form of linear vector summation in the parietal lobe is responsible for our ability to distinguish both the speed and the direction of a moving object—or of the space around us, if we are the moving object.

Beyond the primary sensory areas of the cortex, research has begun to uncover powerful systems in the brain for organizing information in ways that make for an effective response to the environment. In "state control" systems, such as the angle of gaze or attention versus inattention, the "state" exerts an effect on all the information brought together by the system. For example, when we gaze alertly at the road in front of the steering wheel of a car, the parietal lobe's system for peripheral vision creates a "halo" of heightened sensitivity all around the center of our attention, which provides for safe driving.

ATTENTION: A SUBJECT WORTH LOOKING AT

Attention itself has long attracted the interest of those who seek to understand the workings of the brain. What are the essential elements of this hard-to-define state, and what is its underlying physical basis? The great advances in neural imaging of the past 20 years, together with new techniques for observing the living brain at work and refinements in the experimental use of the alert, behaving monkey, offer new ways of studying attention. These new methods have also enhanced the value of behavioral studies by revealing some of their physiological context.

In the view of Michael Posner, of the University of Oregon, psychologists (including Posner) have found it useful in recent years to apply some of the thinking and methods developed for exploration of the visual system to the study of attention.

Our current understanding of attention can be assessed under several headings, which are similar to the areas reviewed by David Hubel for visual perception: the anatomy of the brain structures that appear to be involved; the neural circuitry that makes possible the phenomenon of attention; various developments in the brain after birth that are required for attention; and pathologies, whether injury or disease, that interfere with attention.

THE ANATOMY OF ATTENTION

Positron emission tomography has done much in recent years to change general ideas about the anatomy of mental functions. In particular, PET scans have shown rather distinct localization of the mental operations involved in a task such as "word processing." Under that general heading, it seems at first that many parts of the brain are active, but depending on the specific kind of processing required, activity appears highly focused in one or two areas. PET images of changes in blood flow to discrete areas of the brain (indicative of changes in activity) make it clear that simply showing the experimental subject the written form of a word, and requiring no overt response, activates mainly the visual areas, in the occipital lobe. In PET imaging studies carried out by Posner and Marcus Raichle (discussed in part in Chapter 3), subjects were shown groups of letters that conformed to English rules of construction but did not form a word in English; these nonwords, as well as authentic English words, tended to activate a portion of the left occipital lobe that does not respond to mere strings of consonants or to strings of graphic forms that resemble letters.

This portion of the left occipital lobe is also known to be associated with the brain's system for attention. Patients with "parietal lobe syndrome," described earlier, show a particular effect of parietal injury in their attempts to process words or letter strings shown to them on a screen. If the lesion is in the right parietal lobe, they tend not to notice the first three or four letters of a nonword—that is, those at the left end of the string. But when the letters form a recognizable English word, patients can retrieve it, although they may have difficulty identifying particular letters on the side of the word opposite the site of their injury. Michael Posner, together with Steven Peterson of the Washington University School of Medicine in St. Louis, considers this evidence for a pathway from the parietal lobe (or what they call the "posterior attention system" because of its housing toward the back of the head) to the visual areas of the occipital lobe. (In some other forms of attention, such as planning or mental representation, a number of studies have shown that the frontal lobes play a more important role.) Computer models are being developed to explain how information may be exchanged between the visual system and the posterior attention system.

Despite all it can offer researchers in neuroscience, PET imaging is not ideal for studies of changeable mental states such as attention, because it is not highly time dynamic. It takes about 40 seconds to gather the information from which a PET image is made. Fluctuations of activity within that period will not register in the image; a shift of visual attention, which is accomplished in well under a second, would be invisible. Consequently, behavioral studies of patients with lesions in this area, as well as in a couple of other sites in the midbrain that appear specialized for visual attention, have helped to fill in the picture.

From this work has emerged the finding that a shift of visual attention entails at least two steps: first disengaging the attention from one spot and then bringing it to bear on another location. It appears that the parietal lobe is important in the first step and the midbrain is more active in the second.

NEURAL CIRCUITRY OF AN ATTENTION SYSTEM

The division of labor described above, with one region of the brain responsible for disengaging attention and another for refocusing it, suggests an important distinction between the *source* of an attentional effect and the *site* of its operation. To investigate this possibility, researchers have used electroencephalographic recordings from the scalp during a task in which subjects had their attention drawn to a particular location. The EEG clearly records increases in activity when the subject's attention reaches the target location, as well as slow-wave activity preceding this stage, which presumably indicates disengagement of attention from a previous location. Such methods, which are quite precise as to time and levels of activity, can be combined fruitfully with PET scans or magnetic resonance images to show both the anatomy of interest and time-sensitive readings of activity; researchers then have the means to trace and confirm the circuitry that is thought to be involved in visual attention tasks. Electrical recordings from single cells in alert monkeys, made while the animals' attention was drawn to particular locations, offer another form of information that can be compared with data from PET images and electrode recordings from the scalp in humans.

The posterior attention system apparently is specialized to respond to location in space rather than to other cues such as color or shape or motion. In an experiment in which subjects were asked to attend to these kinds of cues, PET scans showed a distinct pattern of activity, outside the primary visual cortex, associated with each kind of cue. When the target was uncertain, the scans revealed activity in the middle area of the frontal lobe, suggesting the existence of an anterior attention system as well. However, location in space is still the only known visual-attention cue for which the brain has developed exclusive circuitry.

DEVELOPING PATHWAYS IN INFANCY AND CHILDHOOD

The PET studies described earlier that show a specific region of the brain for processing the visual form of words have particular significance for studies of the brain's development. The reading of words is a learned skill that usually does not appear until about 5 years of age. This means that studies of development must take into account the remarkable fact that several years after birth the human brain develops an entirely new visual capacity within the occipital lobe—namely, the ability to recognize the written forms of words in a language (see Plate 7). This new ability presumably entails an important reorganization of the visual system.

To understand how brain development may best be studied in human infants, researchers such as Michael Posner have used the formation of the posterior attention system as a working model. During the first year of life, the six layers of cells that form the visual cortex develop in a definite order, from the deepest layer (closest to the core of the brain) to the most superficial (closest to the surface of the skull). The sequence of development is important because new pathways develop as different layers of the visual system mature. These pathways foster the rapid transmission of signals, perhaps between two areas that before had been connected less directly.

Mark Johnson, of the psychology department at Carnegie Mellon, postulates that at about 1 month of age the human brain develops a pathway that allows an infant to fix his or her eyes on one stimulus and not be distracted by other events at the periphery. This is essentially an inhibitory pathway, because it prevents stimulation by everything but the main target. Studies of laminar development in the brain, which base their work on a large collection of autopsy data assembled over many years, appear to support this idea, as does an interesting marker in infant behavior. From about 1 to 4 months of age, infants practice what is known as "obligatory looking"—that is, once their attention is drawn to a visual target, they seem unable to look away, often remaining fixed on that one target until they become overexcited or begin to cry. After about 4 months (as the posterior attention system matures), they acquire an ability to disengage their attention and are freer to shift their eyes from one object of interest to another.

Working from the adult state back to early development, Michael Posner and his colleagues have traced the origin of another useful element in the posterior attention system: a capacity that inhibits one's eyes from returning to a previous location. Clearly, it is more efficient, when searching for a visual target, not to look in locations that have already been searched. But this "inhibition of return" does not arise from conscious reasoning; instead, it takes form as a specific inhibiting pathway in the brain. The period of its development, between about 3 and 6 months of age, is also when most of the components of this attention system begin to take root.

Such "marker" behaviors as the 1-month-old's obligatory looking or the 3-month-old's tendency to return his eyes to an earlier site are a great help to researchers, who use them as guideposts in the study of development. It is thus possible to investigate, for instance, whether the growth and elaboration of this attention system can be correlated with other maturing abilities, such as the regulation of emotion. The capacity of an infant to be soothed—to shift emotional state under influence from the environment—is one example of a developmental advance that takes place concurrently with some of the early groundwork for the visual attention system.

PATHOLOGY IN THE ATTENTION SYSTEM AND BEYOND

The case files of illnesses and injuries to the brain that interfere with attention systems contain many curious observations (such as the disavowal of parts of one's body mentioned earlier). In these kinds of cases, the symptom makes its appearance on the side opposite the brain hemisphere that is injured. The location of such injuries is often the parietal lobe, and the system most affected by them is the posterior attention system, which is sensitive to location in space.

Meanwhile, the anterior attention system presents its own intriguing patterns of activity. The area of interest here is a little further forward than the site of the posterior attention system, in the middle part of the frontal lobes at a ridge in the brain called the cingulate gyrus. This portion of the brain shows high levels of activity, for example, on PET scans, when subjects in experiments are presented with written words and asked not merely to recognize them but to make some active response, such as saying the words aloud. The cingulate gyrus is also the most active part of the brain (as measured by PET scans of cerebral blood flow) in the well-known psychological phenomenon known as the Stroop effect. The test for this consists of color names that are shown to the subject as written words, but with each word written in a color different from what it says: the word "blue" appears in red, "yellow" in brown, "red" in green, and so on (see Plate 8). When asked to name the color of the ink, most subjects find it all but impossible to override the word they see in favor of the color itself. The very strong activation of the anterior attention system appears to be associated with the compulsion to favor the recognition of the written word over the recognition of color.

Such evidence for the functions of the anterior attention system have led Posner and other researchers to wonder whether defects in this information-coordinating system might also be involved in schizophrenia. Several studies have noted that schizophrenic patients tend to focus on the left side of objects and that they have difficulty shifting attention to the right visual field. Both these signs suggest a dysfunction in the left hemisphere, in an area that is also involved with the processing of language—not that schizophrenic patients as a group show difficulties with language per se, but it is possible that some impairment in the way the brain handles language stimuli could contribute to the disturbances of thought that are characteristic of schizophrenia. Another familiar feature of schizophrenia is the "alien hand sign," in which the patient believes that his hand, although still attached to him, is controlled by an alien power; this is reminiscent of the "neglect" syndrome (discussed earlier) that arises from defects in the posterior attention system. Here, however, the patient still recognizes the hand as his own but imputes the control and direction of its actions to another mind.

One other system for attention seems from early evidence to involve the frontal lobe of the right hemisphere. Injury in this area appears to cause difficulty in so-called vigilance tasks: monitoring a visual (or auditory) field over a long time while on the lookout for rather subtle or infrequent signals. Interestingly, scanning shows that the right frontal cortex is highly active during such tasks but the anterior cingulate gyrus is quite inactive—in fact, it operates below its baseline level of activity. But when the experiment is changed so that the signals become more frequent, the cingulate gyrus increases its participation. This pattern suggests to Posner and others that activity of the vigilance network might effectively inhibit the anterior cingulate gyrus, allowing targets—when they occur—to have ready access to higher levels of attention.

The phenomenon of attention—or the full assortment of mental activities that can be collected under the term "attention"—represents a fine opportunity for research in the Decade of the Brain, because it is terrain on which the cognitive sciences, with their descriptions of processes at the mental level, can join with the anatomical explorations and interpretations of neurobiology. Most alluring for the long term is the prospect that as more becomes known about the anatomical structures and neural circuitry that underlie attention in all its forms, researchers will ultimately be able to resolve a question that curious minds have pondered for a long time: just what goes on in the brain, at a physical level, to account for the subjective experiences of the perceiving mind.

ACKNOWLEDGMENTS

Chapter 7 is based on presentations by David Hubel, Vernon Mountcastle, and Michael Posner.

8

Learning, Recalling, and Thinking

The brain regulates an array of functions necessary to survival: the action of our five senses, the continuous monitoring of the spatial surround, contraction and relaxation of the digestive muscles, the rhythms of breathing and a regular heartbeat. As the vital functions maintain their steady course without our conscious exertion, we are accustomed to consider the brain as preeminently the organ of *thought*. The brain houses our mind and our memories, and we rely on its information-processing capacities when we set out to learn something new.

But where in the brain can we locate memory or thought itself? Chapter 7 offered some clues about the ways scientific investigation—from the molecular level to studies of the alert, behaving animal—has begun to define in physical terms an abstract quality such as "attention." Similiar techniques and approaches are being applied to other mental functions, too, even those as seemingly intangible as learning, remembering, or thinking about the outside world.

Learning and memory, which for many years were considered central problems in psychology, the social sciences, and philosophy, have recently assumed greater importance in the area of neurobiology, itself a confluence of several lines of in-

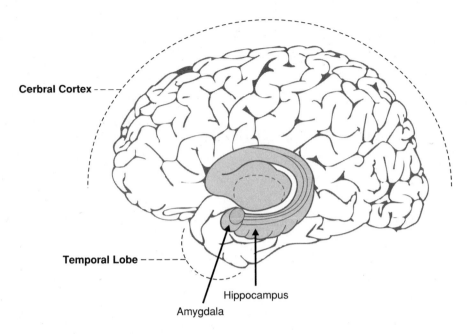

Cerbral Cortex

Temporal Lobe

Hippocampus

Amygdala

FIGURE 8.1.   Most available evidence suggests that the functions of memory are carried out by the hippocampus and other related structures in the temporal lobe. (The hippocampus and the amygdala, nearby, also form part of the limbic system, a pathway in the brain for the signals that underly the emotions.)   It is intriguing to observe that the physical process of laying down a memory by inducing structural changes in individual nerve cells resembles, in some of its features, the sequence of cellular changes in the brain's early growth and development.

vestigation.   Neuroscientific interest in learning and memory has recently increased for two reasons, according to psychiatrist Eric Kandel, a senior scientist in the Howard Hughes Medical Institute at Columbia University.   One reason is the proposal of cellular mechanisms that account for a basic kind of learning and long-term memory.   The model was first identified in the relatively simple nervous systems of the marine snail and the crayfish, but it appears to hold good in the hippocampus of vertebrates as well, where it also may be associated with the formation of long-term memories.

The second reason for a new interest in learning and memory is the evidence accumulating to suggest that mechanisms involved in the structural change in the nervous system that accompanies *learning* may strongly resemble certain important steps in the nervous system's *development*. In other words, the sorts of adjustments among synapses that account for learning may be the same as the "fine-tuning" that occurs while the maturing system is assuming its unique elaborated form. Thus, the biological changes that accompany learning may be seen— in a very schematic way—as an old process put to a new use, or as a specialized way in which the brain continues to "grow" after maturation.

A MOLECULAR ACCOUNT OF LONG-TERM MEMORY

Eric Kandel is best known for his work on the physical basis of learning and memory in the marine snail *Aplysia*. This animal, simple as its nervous system is (most of its 20,000 neurons have been identified by number), nevertheless provides an excellent model for the study of learning and memory, through its "gill withdrawal" reflex. When *Aplysia* perceives something touching its skin, it quickly withdraws both the siphon (a respiratory organ) and the gill, much as a person withdraws a hand from a hot stove without thinking about it. Although this withdrawal is a reflex, it is not completely hard-wired but can be modified by various forms of learning. One such form is sensitization, in which the animal becomes aware of a threatening factor in the environment and to protect itself learns to augment its reflex. The augmented version of the withdrawal reflex can also be maintained in short-term or long-term memory, depending on whether researchers administer the noxious stimulus (the negative reinforcement) only once or twice, or many times within a short period. The two forms of memory can be distinguished not only by their duration—the difference between minutes and days—but also at a molecular level, because it is possible to treat the snail with a chemical compound that interferes with long-term memory but leaves short-term memory unimpaired.

A major set of elements in this reflex are sensory neurons in the siphon skin, which perceive the stimulus; motor neurons in the gill, which contract the muscle and cause the gill to withdraw; and "facilitating neurons," or interneurons, which act on the sensory neurons to enhance their effect. The role of these facilitating neurons has recently become clearer, thanks to observations made from cell cultures, at the simplest level possible: the neurons themselves. A single sensory neuron and a single motor neuron, when implanted in a glass dish with a suitable nourishing culture, form functional interconnections. When a facilitating neuron is added or the cells are exposed to serotonin (the transmitter released by the facilitating neuron), the connection between the sensory and the motor neuron becomes stronger. The connection can last in this enhanced form for more than a day, even up to several weeks, and apparently includes some process of genetic transcription, or expression of part of the nerve cell's DNA.

This genetic transcription produces two results that set long-term memory apart from short-term memory. One is a sort of extension of a short-term effect, in which the potassium channels in the sensory neuron membrane remain closed for a longer time, while the calcium channels remain open. The net effect is that the sensory neuron is more easily excited and releases more neurotransmitter, which in turn activates the motor neuron more strongly. Actually, this effect can be produced on a short-term basis by increased levels of the second-messenger compound cyclic AMP; but after transcription, it is no longer dependent on such a factor and persists even without it. The effect can be disrupted, however, by inhibitors of protein synthesis and RNA synthesis. This constraint establishes that the recording of long-term memories involves not simply a momentary release of neurotransmitters but actual gene expression, with the synthesis of new proteins in the nerve cells themselves.

The new protein products that are synthesized—for example, under the stimulus of a repeated threatening signal—do more than merely reduce the dependence of the sensory neurons on serotonin or cyclic AMP for their activation. As a second transcription event, they induce new growth in certain parts of the sensory neurons themselves. These neurons develop many more presynaptic terminals, the structures through which they release neurotransmitter to the motor neurons; in addition, the number and the surface area of active zones in each presynaptic terminal increase, as does the total number of vesicles, the storage containers for the neurotransmitter. Thus, gene expression appears to build long-term memory out of several effective components, which come together in a formidable array: increased excitability of the sensory neurons, with the protein kinase continuing to work on its own to keep calcium channels open, allowing calcium ions in and more neurotransmitter out; more synapses for conveying signals between sensory and motor neurons; greater numbers of active zones in the synapses; and greater quantities of neurotransmitter contained in the active zones, ready for release. No wonder that memories built of such stuff tend to last awhile.

For closer study, the Kandel laboratory has replicated in cell culture the same conditions that in the living animal lead to protein synthesis and neuronal growth: a motor neuron, a sensory neuron (injected with a fluorescent dye to make imaging possible afterward), and exposure to serotonin repeated four or five times. The results are clear: within several hours, the main axon of the sensory neuron shows an increase in the number of synapses. Exposing the neurons to the second messenger cyclic AMP produces a similiar result. But regardless of whether the facilitating compound is the neurotransmitter or the second messenger, neuronal growth occurs only if a target—a motor neuron—is also present.

The necessary presence of a target was the first similarity that Kandel and his collaborators noticed between the processes of structural change that accompany long-term memory, or learning, and those of development. The observation fit in well, too, with an earlier finding: the fine axonal branches of a sensory neuron in isolation adhere together in fat bundles, but on first contact with a motor neuron the branches tend to separate, each potentially to form its own synapse with the motor neuron. Here, at a mechanical level, is the explanation for a disassembly process that is required prior to the marked increase in synapses that takes place in the presence of serotonin. But in long-term memory, as in development, the presence of the target is necessary—a feature that makes for plasticity, or the all-important ability to change in response to the environment.

To study this learning-related plasticity at the molecular level, Kandel's research group is looking at the proteins that change in level when exposed to serotonin or cyclic AMP (or, in the living animal, to a noxious stimulus). Of the 15 proteins that change, 10 show an increase and 5 show a decrease. The reactions are transient: the levels go up, or down, and back again quite quickly.

Most interesting, in the investigators' view, are the proteins whose response is to decrease in level. Is there a way in which producing *less* of something can figure in a growth process? At a molecular level, the answer can be yes, if the something is an inhibitory factor of some kind. Such an answer may apply in this case, because four of these proteins that have been identified by genetic sequencing turn out to be none other than cell-adhesion molecules of the immunoglobulin type, first discovered by the research team of Gerald Edelman at Rockefeller University.

During development, the proteins apparently play a fundamental role; at least one of them is present at the very first stages, when the fertilized egg begins to divide. In the adult, however, these four proteins appear only in the nervous system, in both sensory and motor neurons. An interesting effect of these cell-adhesion proteins can be demonstrated on an isolated sensory neuron: if an antibody is added that blocks the cell-adhesion effect, the axonal filaments of the neuron start to come apart from their thick bundle and to separate out. The effect is similar to what happens when a sensory neuron is exposed to serotonin in the presence of a target, a motor neuron. This suggests that cell-adhesion molecules can indeed act as an inhibiting factor in particular circumstances. What they inhibit, apparently, is the growth and proliferation of signal-transmitting elements on the axons of sensory neurons.

By this reasoning, the effect of the cell-adhesion molecules would have to be held in abeyance at some point, to allow the sensory neurons to strengthen and increase their synaptic connections with the motor neurons. Perhaps there is even an innate tendency for some neurons, when they are near other target neurons, *always* to have their axons branching and proliferating, always to be seeking to form more synapses. (Indeed, during development, as discussed in Chapter 6, the brain actually forms a great many more synapses than can ever be functional during the animal's lifetime.) The inhibitory action of the cell-adhesion molecules may thus be a crucial factor that keeps neuronal growth somewhat under control, and the temporary inhibition of cell-adhesion molecules in favor of long-term memory may be a single, notable exception to this form of containment. Of course, these results come from painstakingly close study of very simple nervous systems. The degree to which such findings can be extrapolated to the brains of primates, for example, which are many times more complex and which follow different patterns of development, is a matter of lively discussion among researchers in various specialized areas of neuroscience.

One striking aspect of such a system is the ingeniously high level of what, in a person, might be called thriftiness—the degree to which the same materials or biological processes are used and reused, but in novel contexts and to different ends. The protein kinase described earlier, which is dependent on cyclic AMP, appears in many other systems of the body and has various effects; but only in the nervous system, in relation to learning, does it play a role in long-term activation. Likewise, cell-adhesion molecules—better known to researchers for their general role in development—play a rather specialized part in the adult nervous system.

Just as intriguing, from a different perspective, is the evidence for significant common ground between biological mechanisms of learning and the early development of the organism: not only the common use of cell-adhesion proteins (although in different ways) but also the fact that growth in both contexts requires a target. Even the finding that a neurotransmitter such as serotonin is not restricted to moment-by-moment signaling but can actually be a factor that initiates neuronal growth in the case of long-term memory adds to an impression of the two contexts conjoining, with neurotransmitters sometimes acting as growth factors.

THE WORLD IN THE FRONT OF THE BRAIN

Short-term and long-term memory are not the only forms in which the brain stores information. All the time that the five senses are operating, the brain is assembling and sorting perceptions of the outside world, directing some to conscious attention and collecting others into a set of perpetually updated mental representations. Although we may seldom be aware of the full extent of these mental representations, or examine them directly, nevertheless, they hold great importance for our thought processes and our ability to carry out the simplest planned action or predictive step, even something as elementary as following a fast-moving target with our eyes. These mental representations are the data on which we base cognition—our thoughts, ideas, and abstract mental processes.

Animals, too, form complex mental representations of the world, which are shaped by their own brain structure and ecological requirements. For instance, information gathered through the sense of smell undoubtedly plays a much larger role in the mental representations of a dog than in those of a bird, which relies much more on its excellent vision (both in detail and in color) to help it recognize its kin, observe the territories of its rivals, and seek out food and mates. With such differences taken into account, the study of mental representation in animals can help scientists explain similiar processes in humans, particularly if the neurobiology of the animal is also under study or is well known from earlier research.

Mental representation in the monkey, in the form of short-term or working memory, has actually been studied for more than 50 years. The earliest experiments were carried out as delayed-response tests: the monkey was shown a morsel of food being placed in one of two food wells and after a short delay had to open the correct one to claim the food as a reward. The reason for the delay was to force the monkey to rely on an internal mental representation rather than on immediate stimulation—that is, what it saw taking place at that moment. In the rhesus monkey, the area of the brain known to be important for this task is the prefrontal cortex; and in humans, too, homologous areas in the frontal region of the cortex, just behind the forehead, are sites of activity for tasks that test working memory.

Present-day research of this kind with monkeys uses a computer monitor. In such experiments, the animal directs its gaze to the center of the screen. While it keeps its attention fixed on the central spot, a visual target (a light) flashes briefly (for half a second) somewhere else on the screen. The monkey's task (which requires some months of training) is to keep its eyes fixed on the central spot as long as it is lit, and then, when the central spot has been switched off, to move its eyes to the place where the visual target had flashed some seconds before. Clearly, the test calls for working memory: the chances of turning one's eyes to the correct site by a lucky guess are slight, and since the visual target can appear anywhere at all on the screen, in any sequence—not simply location A alternating with location B—there is no possible way to "prepare" the correct response beforehand. A monkey that is practiced in this task can perform with a high degree of accuracy; but when a portion of its principal sulcus is removed by surgery, an animal that was previously proficient performs with no more than 50 percent accuracy.

Given this sharp drop in performance, what is the *nature* of the deficit in the monkey's brain after surgery? Patricia Goldman-Rakic, who directs such investigations at Yale University Medical School, explains that it can be considered a "hole" in the memory—not in vision or in the ability to move the eyes. These faculties show up unimpaired in tests in which the visual target is left on (so that the monkey simply moves its eyes to the target at the appropriate time). Only the ability to guide the response by a mental image (memory) is missing.

Another complementary way of investigating the same topic is to record electrical activity from the brain during a working-memory task. The ideal record in terms of clarity and precision is one obtained from a single neuron, by means of extremely fine microelectrodes. Recordings of this kind have become possible only in the past decade or so; those from Goldman-Rakic's laboratory show several very interesting things. First, the neuron under study, in the prefrontal cortex, holds to a steady level of activity when the target light appears. But it increases its activity sharply once the target light is switched *off* and shows sustained activity during the delay, the interval over which a memory of the target must be maintained. Finally, the neuron's activity rather abruptly returns to a baseline level when the monkey begins its response—that is, when it moves its eyes to the site where the target had been. The neuron thus shows a high level of activity only during the time required to keep the correct spot "in mind" until the moment arrives to respond actively.

A second point of interest from these recordings is that the neurons of this region in the prefrontal cortex each tend to remember one precise location on the screen—and no others. For example, one neuron would respond accurately for targets at a 270-degree rotation from the center but would remain unresponsive to all other locations; another neuron would respond only to targets at a 90-degree rotation. In an analogy with the visual system, the neurons form a "memory field" in much the same way that nerve cells of the occipital lobe form a visual field. The memory field even shows the same cross-brain pattern that is traced by many signals: neurons oriented to the memory of stimuli that appeared in the right visual field predominate in the left hemisphere, and those oriented to the memory of stimuli presented in the left visual field predominate in the right hemisphere.

In Goldman-Rakic's words, memory is an added-on feature of the representation system for visual space. Bearing out this interpretation are recordings from trials during which monkeys that were usually accurate made a mistake in their response, moving their eyes to the wrong place. The electrical data show that the particular neurons for that location were not highly active during the delay period, and so they failed to sustain the mental representation.

According to a current view, these neurons are organized in modules rather like the ocular dominance columns of the visual system. Several lines of research have established that the principal sulcus receives a great deal of its information about the outside world from the parietal cortex, which specializes in visual spatial information (as discussed in Chapter 7). The nerve tracts that project from the parietal lobe do in fact form a pattern of columns in the prefrontal cortex that alternates with columns for incoming signals from other regions. As in the visual system, each column is about half a millimeter wide.

These mental representations in the prefrontal cortex are too limited to be directly responsible for an animal's complex behavior. Goldman-Rakic and her colleagues believe that this representational knowledge does guide behavior in collaboration with other areas—particularly the parietal cortex—and that the larger network very probably represents the neural circuitry underlying spatial cognition in monkeys. Different parts of the network, and the connections among them, must be analyzed separately before the ensemble can be well understood as a network. A broad assortment of psychological studies have shown that when people are asked to perform any cognitive task, the prefrontal cortex invariably is activated; what remains to be discerned is which particular subdivisions of the area (visual or auditory or other) are involved. Increasingly specific testing, anatomical examination, and medical imaging of animals and human subjects are the tools that can provide this kind of information.

Meanwhile, noninvasive medical imaging of humans offers opportunities for the direct simultaneous study of physiology and mental functioning. In addition to NMR and PET scans, electroencephalographic studies can be quite useful, recording electrical activity at the scalp with great temporal precision. Recent EEG studies have shown that when a subject performs cognitive or judgment tasks that require keeping something in mind over a short period, a number of areas in the prefrontal cortex are active. When, on occasion, the subject makes an error, it appears that the network as a whole was not engaged.

NEUROTRANSMITTERS AND THE INFORMATION SYSTEM

In addition to the information-processing circuits arranged in neuronal modules and in columns of incoming nerve tracts, the brain is replete with other systems of input. In the prefrontal cortex, for example, nerve fibers containing the neurotransmitter dopamine are found in especially high concentration, and researchers have wondered for some time what role dopamine might play in prefrontal circuits of information. The evidence gathered on this point over the past few years has begun to make clear the enormous extent to which dopamine shapes not only our physical functioning in the world but also our ability to process new information, to associate ideas effectively, and even to maintain a sense of well-being in balance with realistic perceptions.

In the human prefrontal cortex, the nerve fibers containing dopamine are not scattered evenly throughout the six cerebral cell layers but are concentrated in the outermost layers and the deep layers—that is, in layers 1, 5, and 6—and are less densely distributed in the middle layers. The cell bodies of these neurons are located relatively far away in the ventral tegmental area, a portion of the brainstem; they preferentially project their fibers to the frontal and prefrontal cortex. In addition, researchers have identified at least two distinct kinds of receptor sites for dopamine, and each has its own pattern in the layers of the cortex. The preponderance of the D-1 receptor fairly matches that of the dopamine-containing fibers: very high in the outermost layers and also considerable in the deep layers. The D-2 receptor, by contrast, shows a lower concentration throughout, with just a mild peak in layer 5.

In a test to see whether interference with the D-1 receptors would have any effect on cognitive function, Goldman-Rakic's research team injected a compound that blocks the D-1 receptor sites in the prefrontal cortex of monkeys trained in the delayed-response test described earlier. About 20 minutes after the injection, the animals showed an impairment of working memory, moving their eyes to the wrong location when the trial included a delay; but they responded correctly in a "sensory-guided" version of the task, in which the target light was left on as a guide. The D-1 receptors thus appear to be implicated in the efficiency of working memory.

A chemical compound developed for use in research that selectively stains neurons in the cerebral cortex bearing D-1 receptor sites has provided the Yale research team with an interesting lead. These neurons have been identified as pyramidal cells, the large principal cells that are the main element of cerebral cortex layer 6. The axons of these cells carry signals to another region—in this case, the thalamus (which plays an important role in the control of movement and forms part of the limbic system).

It appears from electron-microscopy studies that the dopamine receptors on these cells may modulate excitatory synapses, possibly from other pyramidal cells in the same or another region. Therefore, since dopamine acts directly on the output neurons of the prefrontal cortex—which are involved in processing, sorting, and assembling information about the outside world—the dopamine circuits can be considered a physical pathway by which this neurotransmitter can influence cognitive function. With each neuron bearing millions of spines on which dopamine synapses may act, a mechanism of this kind can have a pervasive effect, and even a slight deficiency or excess of dopamine could powerfully alter the ability of many neurons to integrate information from other regions of the brain. Goldman-Rakic and her colleagues are looking closely at the identified dopamine synapses to understand more precisely the mechanism by which dopamine may affect cognition.

The prefrontal cortex, with its importance for cognition, shows a form of dysfunction when tested in patients suffering from schizophrenia. (An often disabling mental illness, schizophrenia interferes with the capacity for logical thought and greatly disturbs the emotions and social behavior; see Chapter 4 for a discussion of current theories about the importance of dopamine levels in schizophrenia.) In experiments calling for cognitive tasks, which normally require the participation of the prefrontal cortex, schizophrenic patients show significantly lower rates of activity in this region of the brain. This does not mean that a disorder as complex and varied in form as schizophrenia can be explained as a simple failure of one part of the brain— particularly since the prefrontal cortex is known to be so richly interconnected with many other regions. But the findings that indicate a less active prefrontal cortex, which have been replicated in numerous studies, fit in well with other evidence suggesting that some dysfunction in a *network* of areas, including the prefrontal cortex, is implicated in schizophrenia.

Studies are under way to probe the state of working memory in schizophrenic patients as a way of learning more about the normal and impaired functioning of the prefrontal cortex. Meanwhile, rhesus monkeys treated in such a way as to mimic some of the deficits characteristic of schizophrenia are also being tested for working memory, thereby allowing more direct study of the neurobiology involved. One of the behavioral deficits that has been experimentally produced in monkeys is the inability to track a fast-moving target with the eyes. The deficit is not based in the visual or motor system; this much is clear, because the monkeys remain able to track targets moving more slowly. Instead, the problem seems to be cognitive, an inability to predict where the target will be in the next fraction of a second. This predictive aspect of eye movements, which falters in schizophrenic patients and in the experimentally treated animals, may well draw on the type of mental representations that the prefrontal cortex is largely occupied in assembling. The research being conducted in animals and humans is mutually helpful, offering the prospect over the next decade of significant advances in a neuroscientific account of the workings of the prefrontal cortex—including a cellular explanation of this area's memory functions. A view shared currently by Goldman-Rakic and many colleagues is that the main function of this greatly enlarged part of the brain, so recently evolved in the primate line, is to guide behavior by means of mental representations of stimuli, rather than by the stimuli themselves. Over the course of primate evolution, the advantages of this mode of mental functioning would have been considerable, greatly expanding the animal's options for varied and complex behavior.

WHAT KIND OF COMPUTER IS THIS?

The types of mental representation discussed above, such as the continuous monitoring of the spatial surround by the parietal lobes, illustrate a vital point that is often overlooked when comparisons are made between the human brain and the computer. The fact is that the human brain—or the brain of many other animals—is solving quite difficult computational problems at every moment, just in seeing, recognizing a voice, or moving in a coordinated fashion on four limbs, or two limbs, or two wings. Most of these problems are so complex that they have yet to be formulated in explicit terms by computer scientists, which is why machines that can perceive and move and communicate as animals do—and perform all these functions at once—are still largely the stuff of science fiction.

If computers are not really brains, what does it mean to call the brain a kind of computer? Terrence J. Sejnowski, whose work at the Salk Institute for Biological Studies in San Diego focuses on computer models of cognition and brain structure, answers this question by pointing to a simple device designed to do one thing optimally, and one thing only: play tic-tac-toe. This "computer," built from electronic Tinkertoys at MIT's Artificial Intelligence Laboratory, is programmed with every possible position in the game. (These have been reduced, through mathematical operations that apply the principle of symmetry, to a subset of about 48.) The positions, each with its one optimal response, are encoded as the computer's memory. When presented with a particular position, the computer matches it to one in its subset and produces the correct response. By contrast, a digital computer would meet the challenge with a set of programmed instructions that it would run through recursively at each move to arrive at the optimal response.

The MIT device does not carry out a string of calculations or algorithms, the kind of task we generally think of a computer performing; instead, what it offers is essentially a "look-up table," with the correct answer precomputed and readily available. To obtain swift access to that answer, however, one must present a problem that exactly matches one of the problems originally encoded in the computer's memory. Beyond that pre-encoded set, the computer cannot provide any correct answer—or even a partial answer—unlike a digital computer, which can be reprogrammed for new problems because of its more general mode of operation. Still, within the realm of its pre-encoded problems and responses, the "look-up table" is extremely fast and effective.

This kind of device, however, requires a great deal of memory, since every significant aspect of each pre-encoded problem must be specified if the match is to be accurate. For the game of tic-tac-toe this is manageable; for chess, with its 10^{40} possible game positions, or for real-life contexts in which the rules are less clear, it is impossible, at least at present. As a practical device, the look-up table is strictly limited. However, the principle of precomputing certain responses and being able to retrieve them with minimal additional effort appears to Sejnowski and others in his field as a likely clue to some of the workings of the brain. True, the abundant memory required by a look-up table was extremely expensive in the first computers and still poses a practical challenge today. But if the amount of memory were tremendously expanded, it would be possible to store many more solutions—in other words, to address many more and different kinds of problems.

It is hardly a revelation at this point that the human brain exhibits just such a tremendous capacity to store information. With somewhere between a hundred billion and a trillion neurons, the human brain already looks fairly impressive—but what really expands its storage capacity far beyond anything we can yet envision on an engineer's drawing board is the brain's proliferation of synapses. Each neuron contains several thousand points at which signals can be transmitted. Even if the brain were to store information at the low average rate of one bit per synapse (in terms comparable to a digital code, the synapse would be either active or inactive), the structure as a whole could still build up vast stores of memory, on the order of 10^{14} bits. Meanwhile, today's most advanced supercomputers command a memory of about 10^9 bits. The human brain, to use Sejnowski's phrase, is memory-rich by comparison.

Of course, organization is crucial to managing such a vast resource, and the brain exhibits this feature at several levels, as discussed throughout this book. Research conducted on the simpler nervous system of invertebrates, as well as on nonhuman primates, other vertebrates, and humans, has indicated how learning brings about structural changes in nerve cells and how the neurons in turn form regions, which take part in networks. The networks are organized into distributed systems, which collaborate with other systems, both sensory and associative, to produce the total working effect.

Memory itself is organized so as to take advantage of these many levels of information: it appears to be arranged along associative paths, by the principle of contiguity. That is, the brain associates bits of information in such a way that we can recall items either on their own or by being "reminded" of them by a cue. The name of an acquaintance may come to mind when needed, or we may search for it under one heading or another: the name sounded like that of another friend, or the person looked like a former co-worker, or the meeting took place at the lunch following a difficult business negotiation. Considering the brain in purely physical terms, researchers have suggested that another form of contiguity may apply as well, that is, the simple proximity that builds up into maps. It may be that neurons close enough to one another to be activated together keep some trace of that contiguity as part of their bit of information.

Just what the memory-forming mechanisms might be, at a physiological level, has long puzzled psychologists as well as neurobiologists. Evidence of several kinds is gathering, however, in support of a model first suggested in 1949 by Donald Hebb, that a memory forms as a result of at least two kinds of activity taking place at a synapse simultaneously. The activities would have to include both the pre- and postsynaptic elements, the neuron transmitting the signal and the one receiving it. Hebb reasoned that the strength of the signal received in the postsynaptic cell would depend on the interaction of many details—the amount of transmitter released, the presence or absence of neuromodulators that affect the postsynaptic cell's excitability, the number of receptor sites on the receiving cell, and other such variables. Whatever the specifics, the underlying principle would be that information is stored as a result of two or more biochemical factors coming together in time, at the same instant, and in space, at the same synapse.

Physical evidence that indirectly supports this model has come recently from Eric Kandel's work with *Aplysia*. Hebb postulated two active elements (the pre- and postsynaptic terminals), but the nervous system in the marine snail appears to include a third element, the facilitating neuron that enhances the excitability of the sensory neuron. The Hebbian principle still applies, however, to the extent that the variables have to meet in time and space at a synapse.

In mammals, an example that conforms even better to the Hebbian model is found in part of the hippocampus of rats. The particular area, designated CA-3, contains about half a million neurons with recurrent connections—in other words, many of their axons lead back into the same population of neurons. Some axons also lead into the adjacent area CA-1. At the synapses in this area, both among CA-3 cells and between CA-3 and CA-1 cells, the neurotransmitter glutamate is released. It binds to two types of receptors: at one type of receptor site the glutamate slightly lowers the excitability threshold of the neuron, but at the other the binding of glutamate does not in itself affect the cell. Another simultaneous event is required: depolarization of the receiving cell, perhaps by other synapses. When this occurs together with the binding of glutamate, the cell membrane becomes momentarily permeable to ions—particularly calcium ions, which are important for bringing about persistent changes in the structure of the cell.

This receptor system illustrates the principle of contiguity outlined by Hebb: the binding of glutamate to a particular kind of receptor site and the depolarization of the postsynaptic cell must occur simultaneously, or at least within the same 20 to 50 thousandths of a second, for calcium ions to enter the cell and induce structural changes.

ASSEMBLING A BRAIN IN THE LABORATORY

Hebbian synapses have also been demonstrated in another kind of laboratory, where computer scientists and engineers have built them into a computer chip. The device is a simple one, with only 16 synapses, but it performs Hebbian learning quite efficiently, at the rate of a million times per second. Newer chips have already been developed to represent more realistic neurons, with many thousands of synapses; and technology to represent the connections between such neurons will make the assembly of something more nearly resembling a working brain a little easier to envision. Such a device will have to combine analog signals, like those propagated within neurons, and digital signals, the off or on impulses transmitted from one neuron to another. It will not be simply a larger, or even an unbelievably faster, version of today's familiar computer.

An artificial brain of this kind could be invaluable for further research along two main lines. For one, it could be set to work on some of the more difficult problems in an emerging field that might be called "artificial perception": problems of computer vision and of speech recognition that can be delineated by current devices but that cannot be resolved by them in a practical way. For a second main line of research, this kind of artificial brain can offer an advanced testing ground for neuroscientists' ideas about how the brain functions. Theoretical models of memory, in particular, cannot be tested adequately on a digital-computer simulation of a few hundred model neurons, because the living brain works on such an enormously larger scale. But a computerized circuit of several million model neurons, with information circulating in real time, could yield a whole new order of information about such circuits in the living animal.

The field of artificial perception already boasts chips developed at the California Institute of Technology that are capable of much of the sensory processing performed just outside the brain by the retina, for example, and by the cochlea, the spiral passage of the inner ear whose hair cells respond to vibrations by sending impulses to the auditory nerve. Now in development as well are chips to simulate some of the functions of the visual cortex; others, with some of the memory-storing capacity of the hippocampus, are being scaled up, closer to the dimensions of a living system.

But more time and knowledge are needed to produce a device that can successfully mimic the information processing of the five senses and of short-term and long-term memory, and that can, moreover, integrate these systems into a unit that functions as a whole with respect to the outside world. This is not to say that progress has not occurred: early computers of the 1950s carried out only a few thousand instructions per second (a speed matched by today's pocket calculators), whereas the fastest of the supercomputers in use today can perform billions of operations per second. Still, this rate of processing, at 10^9 or so operations per second, is far from that of the human brain, in which an estimated 10^{14} synapses are each active about 10 times per second—giving a total of 10^{15} operations per second.

An interesting constraint that confronts computer designers who work with the current top speeds is the simple, unchanging limitation posed by the speed of light. Signals simply cannot be transmitted faster than about 1 foot per billionth of a second (10^{-9}, the speed of light); to achieve the effect of speeds higher than this, the computer must be reduced in size to less than a cubic foot. This reduction is made possible by duplicating the central processor many times, even thousands of times, within the same computer, so that signals have less distance to travel. Even so, extrapolating from the recent rate of increase and from today's highest known speeds of computer processing, Terrence Sejnowski estimates that an artificial device approximating the human brain cannot be expected before at least the year 2015.

This prediction should not be considered discouraging—far from it. For such a project to be within sight at all is the clearest possible sign of the progress of neuroscience, gaining impetus as it does from an increasing number of fields that are related in some way to its investigations. Now not only the biological sciences, medicine, biochemistry, pharmacology, and psychology have an interest in improving our understanding of the brain's functioning; the computer sciences, physics, and mathematics also contribute to such models and stand to gain much from their continued exploration and testing. And along the way toward the assembly of a fully functioning artificial brain, it should become increasingly possible to construct devices that satisfactorily replicate *some* of the principles at work in the human brain. Although the devices probably would not resemble a brain in their material form any more than an airplane resembles a bird, they will be successful if they can show some of the brain's operating principles adapted to their own form, just as an airplane carries out, in mechanical translation, some of the aerodynamic principles of natural flight.

THE BENEFITS OF AN ARTIFICIAL BRAIN

Of course, the brain cannot ever be completely characterized in terms of a computer because in addition to all its computing faculties it possesses the properties of a biological organ in a living system. But, points out Gerald Edelman of the Neurosciences Institute at Rockefeller University, computers can indeed do something that, until recently, only a brain could do: they can carry out logical functions. Today, a computer can address any challenge or problem that can be described in a logical formula. This still leaves unexplored vast areas of human experience, such as perception; but as described earlier in this chapter, computer and mathematical modeling on one side, and more detailed neurobiological examination on the other side, are making inroads in this area too.

Edelman and his colleagues have used an approach they call synthetic neural modeling to build an automaton that is able to explore its environment by simulated vision and touch; moreover, it can categorize objects on the basis of its perceptions, and its responses draw on previous experiences with similar objects. Darwin III (the third generation of its kind) is a robot whose nervous system is built of about 50,000 cells of different types. The signals transmitted at its approximately 640,000 synaptic junctions enable Darwin III to control the functioning of its one eye and its multijointed arm. In analogy with the way living brains enter the world, Darwin III has no specific information built into its systems about the objects it may encounter in its environment. The nervous system is pre-encoded only to the extent that the devices for perception are made to detect certain features, such as light or movement or rough texture.

An important principle of Darwin III's nervous system is that the strength of the synaptic connections can increase selectively with greater activity when that activity leads to an adaptive end. What is "adaptive" for Darwin III is defined by arbitrary values built into its programming. For example, the built-in principle that light is "better" than no light serves to direct and refine the system's eye movements toward a target. Just as in living neurons, the enhanced connection provides a stronger response the next time that particular neural pathway is active.

This selective strengthening of connections is reminiscent of the competition among synapses in the developing brain (as discussed in Chapter 6). Together with the ability to categorize, it means that the system can produce behaviors that we commonly call "recognition," for instance, or "association." At present, Darwin III can turn its head to track a moving object with its eye; it can extend its arm to trace the contours of an object; and, alternatively, if the stimulus is noxious, it can swat the object away. In all these responses the system shows increasing accuracy with practice, as the relevant synapses are strengthened. Eventually, such a system should be able to teach itself to apply both visual and motor abilities to a complex task—for instance, distinguishing a particular object or kind of object, and picking it out with the arm from among many others.

Although Darwin III cannot represent the nervous system of living animals in a highly detailed way, its synapses and circuits provide a much-needed testing ground for ideas about what takes place inside the real thing that makes those 3 pounds of semisoft tissue the most complex information-processing system ever known. Perhaps computers can never be brains in the full sense of serving as the nervous center of a biological system, but they can be designed with increasing success to carry out some of the functions that are routinely managed by a living brain. Gerald Edelman, like Terrence Sejnowski, believes that the prospects for building more complex "perception machines" are good—and the benefits in both intellectual and economic terms will be enormous. Most important of all would be the expanded opportunities for an understanding of higher brain functions—those that make us human—to be gained by using the computer not so much as a model of the brain, but as a tool for exploring it.

ACKNOWLEDGMENTS

Chapter 8 is based on presentations by Gerald Edelman, Patricia Goldman-Rakic, Eric Kandel, and Terrence Sejnowski.

9

Sizing Up the Promise

How can neuroscience best fulfill its rich promise in the Decade of the Brain? One of the events of the symposium sponsored in July 1990 by the Institute of Medicine and the National Institute of Mental Health was a panel discussion that focused on the questions "What needs to be done?" and, more pragmatically, "What can be done?" Led by Joseph B. Martin, dean of the School of Medicine at the University of California, San Francisco, the panel consisted of half a dozen spokesmen from government, academia, industry, and the private sponsorship of research, all sectors committed to advancing neuroscience.

The question "What needs to be done?" calls up a vigorous response from the neuroscience community. The needs are great: with some form of brain illness or mental disorder likely to strike one in every eight Americans, and with as many as 1,000 different dysfunctions of the brain thought to be determined at least in part by genetic makeup, it is clear that this field of knowledge holds great potential to alleviate illness and suffering, through the clinical tools of diagnosis and treatment and through genetic analysis. The imperative to use our cur-

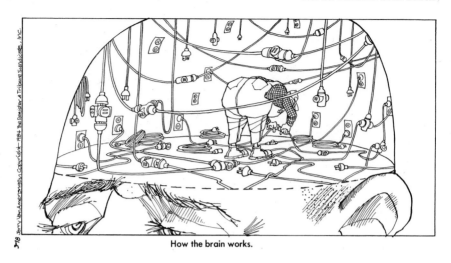

How the brain works.

FIGURE 9.1. Policy decisions concerning the support of research in neuroscience are at least as complex as the scientific field itself. Source: Jerry Van Amerongen, 1984©. Reprinted with special permission of King Features Syndicate, Inc.

rent knowledge to these ends, and to continue extending that knowledge, is hardly in doubt.

It is in response to the question "What can be done?" that expert opinions diverge, because neuroscience faces far greater opportunities in research than there are resources to carry them out. Research questions that could scarcely have been conceived 10 or 15 years ago, much less investigated fruitfully, can now be explored. The theoretical context—in neurology, in molecular biology, and in genetics—is in place, and the technology—whether in cloning, magnifying, or imaging with pinpoint accuracy—is available. But the likelihood that such investigations can be sustained over a long period is less assured than in the past. True, the strain on resources in neuroscience research can be seen as a measure of success, both in attracting a generation of talented workers and in yielding many lines of inquiry worthy of their attention. But such success must seem a mixed blessing, at best, to the young researcher who hears that these days less than one in four grant proposals may be funded. (Many more than this are of excellent quality and are actually approved, but simply do not rank high enough on the list to receive funding in a time of limited resources.)

DEFINING THE FIELD OF INQUIRY

The scope of neuroscience is virtually limitless—it is nothing less than the seeking by the human brain to understand itself. Small wonder that the field draws on other scientific disciplines, some closely related and others that might at first appear more distant: cellular and molecular biology, behavioral sciences, and computational science, but also quantum mechanics and the new field of chaos theory. (This last may soon offer models for some of the processes that take place in integrating information—a task at which the human brain excels.) In addition, neuroscience research in the future will depend more on sophisticated technologies for observing the brain at work and for recording and sorting the flood of information that can be obtained. Computerized databases of neural circuitry—an open archive of the pathways and connections of any of the brain's 100 billion nerve cells—could provide answers and save time for countless research projects. The development of such tools has been proposed by a committee of the Institute of Medicine.

Within neuroscience itself, research progresses by means of loops, or back-and-forth exchanges between areas of inquiry that are mutually informative. One of the essential loops occurs between macrobiology and molecular biology; it goes from sophisticated measures of behavior to the precise identification of the nerve cells that underlie a particular movement or perception or memory, and then back again to the animal's behavior. In this connection, it is clear that curtailing the macrobiological studies, under pressure from nonscientists to abandon animal testing, works to the detriment of the whole enterprise; for without behavioral studies as a way of checking theories in the "real world," cellular or molecular explanations of how the brain works can advance only a short way before sinking into conjecture. Likewise, in the examination of the human brain, the loop between research and clinical practice means that each side provides the other with the tools to proceed further. The study of schizophrenia is a notable example. Clinicians—psychiatrists and psychologists—have assembled the many forms and clinical signs of this disorder under a single heading; molecular biologists and geneticists are tracing patterns of inheritance, and neuroscientists have begun to uncover some of the physical abnormalities of the brain that are associated with schizophrenia. This research feeds back into clinical practice by offering more precise criteria for diagnosis.

Because neuroscience spans so many fields of investigation, the funding for such research must also be broadly based. In the United States, the federal government disburses about $8 billion annually to support biomedical research, largely through the Public Health Service of the Department of Health and Human Services, which comprises the various National Institutes of Health and the Alcohol, Drug Abuse, and Mental Health Administration. Federal funds also support related projects that are carried out for the Food and Drug Administration and even the Department of Energy. Of this total, about $1.2 billion goes to support research in neuroscience. The Public Health Service is particularly strong in research on mental and addictive disorders, funding almost 85 percent of the nation's efforts in these areas.

The federal government's support of brain research is roughly equalled by funding from the private sector—that is, industry, private foundations, voluntary health agencies, and not-for-profit research institutions. Most notable in this last category is the Howard Hughes Medical Institute, which disburses more than $200 million annually for basic biomedical research at about 50 universities around the country; in 1990, it directed about $35 million toward research in neuroscience. Other private foundations that are not devoted exclusively to biomedicine nevertheless contribute substantial sums to basic research: in 1985, the Alfred P. Sloan Foundation gave $9 million, the John D. and Catherine T. MacArthur Foundation $12 million, and the Pew Charitable Trusts $21 million. In addition, a great many smaller foundations support research on a specific disease or disorder; such foundations often begin as one family's personal response to affliction.

As the costs of research have increased, the role of industry as a significant source of support has also grown, making it second only to the federal government. Although the pharmaceutical industry, for example, directs nearly 80 percent of its research funds toward product development, it is also farsighted enough to fund both basic and applied research. For example, FIDIA, the fourth-largest pharmaceutical company in Italy, reinvests 25 percent of its profits each year in a combination of basic and clinical research specifically in neuroscience. In the United States, the pharmaceutical industry as a whole spent about $860 million in 1988 to support research on the central nervous system and sense organs; this figure amounted to almost 15 percent of total sales for that year.

SCIENCE EDUCATION AND SCIENCE ADVOCACY

At the same time that neuroscience is launched on what could be its most rewarding and exciting decade yet, another challenge is taking shape outside the laboratory—and researchers would be wise to tackle it promptly. This challenge is found in a paradoxical and widespread attitude toward science: the general public depends increasingly on scientific research, and at the same time expresses a growing mistrust of science and its practitioners. Secretary of Health and Human Services Louis Sullivan has said that the general public—particularly the young—often describe science with "four C's": costly, cruel, corrupt, and closed. For science to bear such an image—even if it is based on ignorance—is unaffordable, by any calculations. Not only the necessity for public support of research but also the steadily growing need to draw bright young minds into the field calls for supporters of science to correct these misperceptions with all due speed.

The proper tool to bring about this change is, of course, science education. This can take many forms in addition to what goes on in a classroom—for example, a corporate-sponsored exhibit on the history of neuroscience. And in the mass media, even something as superficial as including scientists among the characters in everyday television programs could contribute toward drawing young people into the field, if the portrayals could be made to avoid the stereotype of the mad scientist or its modern variants (cold and unfeeling, or earnest and unattractive).

Frederick Goodwin, of the Alcohol, Drug Abuse, and Mental Health Administration, speaks of "frayed edges around what we used to call scholarship": the production of data has taken researchers' time away from reaching out to maintain the public understanding of science, from making the best information available to those who teach science in the primary and secondary schools, and even from explicitly conveying the values of science to those who are considering a career in research.

The image of the profession has also suffered from recent examples of misconduct in science. At the same time, formal handling of some cases of misconduct has brought about a clash of cultures, in which an adversarial system—the law—is asked to rule on principles and practices of science that have been shaped largely by consensus.

Too often, senior scientists pressed by the multiple demands of high-level research have less time available than they would like for serving as mentors. The current climate may reflect a widespread tendency to pay attention to immediate crises and leave long-term problems to take care of themselves. But this national preference for investing in the short term, says Goodwin, will provide very poorly for the future of science. The federal government should take more of a hand in helping to prepare the next generation in science, and to this end it may be appropriate to fund some of the professional associations or groups that engage in educating the public about science.

The small foundations may be the best instruments for presenting the workings of science to the public: they have scientific understanding, motivation, and energy in abundance, combined with resources less extensive than those the federal government can allot to research, but nevertheless substantial. Thomas Langfitt, of the Pew Charitable Trusts, believes that foundations might well be interested in forming better coalitions with the scientific community to convey the value of science, particularly biomedical research, to the nation at large. But such a message cannot be simply stated. It requires careful presentation, because it risks disillusioning a public that may be too anxious about questions of health and well-being to allow plenty of time for thorough research. A basic understanding of the nature of science, inculcated from earliest schooling, could help the public develop more realistic expectations of the scientific enterprise.

THE FEDERAL GOVERNMENT AS SPONSOR OF RESEARCH

Of all the institutions dedicated to seeing the Decade of the Brain fulfill its promise, the federal government—as befits the largest sponsor—is pursuing the greatest variety of activities. Within the Department of Health and Human Services, the Public Health Service has singled out four areas of involvement. First is the ongoing support of investigator-initiated biomedical research (as opposed to research assigned by contract) throughout the country. Many of the grant programs of NIH and ADAMHA, in particular, are directed toward investigations in neuroscience.

Second, the federal government is in the best position to amass the resources for science projects of all sizes and to coordinate major efforts with those of other countries, as is being done for the human genome project. This long-term multinational initiative, which some researchers have feared might overshadow other projects in biomedicine in terms of public support or funding, is beginning to show its usefulness for numerous research fields outside genetics. For example, it is clear that neuroscience has an interest in the mapping and sequencing of the human genome, since as many as 1,000 of the roughly 3,500 diseases and syndromes known to be carried in the genetic code affect the brain or the nervous system.

A third, essential function of the Public Health Service is to clarify the priorities for federally sponsored research in an era of deficit budgets. The fourth function may be the most urgent: developing ways to nurture the next generation of neuroscientists. The Public Health Service is considering incentives for schools and research centers to recruit bright students into the field, and new ways to increase the overall scientific literacy of the public. James Mason, in the Department of Health and Human Services, urges scientists to use the Decade of the Brain to its fullest potential in this regard. The decade offers opportunities on all sides: for conveying the excitement of working in neuroscience and the value of this work to the nation's health; for raising public awareness of the dangers posed by avoidable injuries of the brain and spinal cord in accidents, by substance abuse, and by the presence of neural toxins in a polluted environment; and, as we come increasingly to appreciate the complexity of the brain, for nourishing the mind as well, by providing every child with a good basic education.

In the executive branch, the White House Office of Science and Technology Policy (OSTP) has responsibility for coordinating the many efforts and initiatives that make up the Decade of the Brain. One necessary item is a comprehensive federal plan for supporting research in neuroscience, and to that end OSTP has assembled a working group that includes representatives from government agencies involved in a broad spectrum of brain research. The group also includes representatives from the departments of commerce, education, and state, because the implications from brain research touch on so many areas, even those as far afield as technology transfer, international efforts to promote science, and global competitiveness. A 10-year national research plan for neuroscience would lay the groundwork for the federal government's organization of research funding well into the future.

The activities of the Decade of the Brain are directed mainly toward two groups: the public, with the goal of increasing science literacy, and the scientific community, with a long-term research plan as the objective. The OSTP working group has selected eight areas of research for special attention: addiction; aging; development; education, learning, and memory; human behavior and mental disorders; communications and sensory disorders; brain and spinal cord injury; and rehabilitation and restoration of function. The OSTP group will use these eight areas as the base for a detailed research plan for the decade, in consultation with federal research agencies, the academic community, and voluntary health organizations. OSTP itself will act as a clearinghouse for resources and efforts from all sectors, fulfilling its traditional role while also contributing to what White House science adviser Allan Bromley calls "one of the most important initiatives that the federal government is undertaking in science and technology in this decade."

A long-term plan may be especially suitable for neuroscience, where the complexity of questions to be addressed and the intricacy of the systems under study can make the research trail very long. Many senior scientists, who must not only plan their own projects but also advise students proposing to enter the field, would like to see stable (or growing) levels of funding from one year to the next. As one participant at the panel discussion remarked, "Scientists like prediction"—but even a scientific prediction is only as good as the information on which it is based. The need for more farsighted planning in neuroscience is gaining recognition around the world, as other countries—Italy and Canada thus far—consider their own version of the Decade of the Brain.

PRIVATE INDUSTRY AND PRIVATE FOUNDATIONS

The unusual but highly effective alliance of industry and private foundations makes up a solid base of support for neuroscience. Tightly focused programs sponsored by industry have long been effective. To date, these have been mostly intramural programs—within a company's own research facilities—but the time is ripe to begin building cooperative extramural programs with the academic, scientific, and medical communities. For some clinical trials, these alliances are already in place. Industry contributes in these cases by continuing to develop sharper measures of efficacy, more powerful theoretical models, and more informative procedures; it also supports clinical research training within the medical community, industry's irreplaceable partner in therapeutic development. FIDIA Pharmaceutical Corporation, for example, is considering whether to establish a number of fellowships for clinical research training in neurology, similar to the corporation's support for basic research.

Industry can also help substantially in the area of communications. Alberto Grignolo, president of FIDIA, identifies three target audiences, each needing a distinct message. To the government, industry should carry the message that it is vital to continue to invest in biomedical research—particularly neuroscience research. To the academic community, industry needs to convey its interest in collaborating on the best possible research and in translating knowledge into therapeutic advances. And to the public, industry should clearly announce and reiterate that better diagnoses and new treatments depend on continued investment in both basic and applied research.

In contrast to the broad reach of industry, the aims of private foundations tend to be more narrowly focused. A foundation with a research budget of, say, several million dollars per year for neuroscience finds itself in an interesting niche. Clearly, it cannot compete with the federal government in funding worthy projects, nor can it necessarily command the expertise and resources needed to run an effective peer-review system for selecting those projects. What such a foundation does instead is create (or skillfully discover) those research initiatives that are of high quality but that are unlikely to receive funding through conventional channels. Thomas Langfitt, of the Pew Charitable Trusts, says there are two likely reasons a promising application for funding might be turned down by NIH or another federal research agency. First, the research may seem too risky—often simply because it is at too early a stage for the outcome to be clearly predictable. Second, it may be too interdisciplinary, that is, not strictly within the bounds of one scientific field or another and thus difficult to evaluate. Yet if research of this kind can obtain support from a private foundation at an early stage, the work may well go on to win approval from a government research agency later on.

With this reasoning, the Pew Trusts have recently launched two initiatives for funding in neuroscience. One is aimed at bringing basic research and clinical practice closer together in neuroscience; the other is designed to foster cross-disciplinary thinking—that is, to encourage a wide variety of traditionally unrelated fields (cognitive psychology, primate behavior, computer science, linguistics, philosophy) to contribute to neuroscience and to be enriched by it in turn. The Pew Trusts have also awarded grants to laboratories for the development of cell lines of neural tissue—an emerging need among research departments of medical institutions.

The cross-disciplinary initiative, the McDonell–Pew Cognitive Neuroscience Program, focuses on research and training, awarding funds to research centers at several institutions and also disbursing a number of smaller grants each year. This program makes a particular effort to enlist researchers who are already well under way in their field—graduate students or postdoctoral fellows—and who know they will need to become familiar with at least one other discipline to pursue their line of interest. The exchange thus fostered should help to give cognitive neuroscience the broadest possible base for exploring the subtle, intricate relationship between the human mind and its physical counterpart, the brain.

A small private foundation can effectively support neuroscience by promoting research on just one or two disorders. The National Alliance for Research on Schizophrenia and Depression (NARSAD) is an example of this approach; the alliance currently funds several dozen investigators, primarily in their early years of research, awarding more than $3.5 million in grants. Applications for grants are not as complex as those required by federal funding agencies but nevertheless undergo first-rate peer review, thanks to a number of eminent scientists who donate their time. Despite its limited resources, the alliance is clearly meeting a need: its small-grants program attracts between 600 and 700 applications per year. A foundation oriented toward public relations, such as the David Mahoney Institute for the Decade of the Brain, may favor a broader approach. This not-for-profit group was founded by nonscientists, with an advisory board drawn from science, business, and the media. David Mahoney sees the institute's mission as helping to "coordinate, orchestrate, and unify the efforts of all interested parties in support of the Decade of the Brain"—in essence, an institute for public education.

A FUTURE RICH WITH CHALLENGES

Explaining neuroscience to the public poses special difficulties. For one thing, in any specific area of research, the complexity of the system under study is hard to take in. We cannot readily envision 10^{11} nerve cells, even when we are told we carry them around inside our head—or perhaps *especially* when we are told this. In addition, many people already have quite definite ideas about how their mind works, ideas in which values such as free will and independence of action may play a large part. When a scientific explanation appears to overlook these values and presents instead an account that is highly complex and based on invisible principles (or invisibly small molecules), it may well meet with some resistance.

But not all the odds are stacked against neuroscience. An important human factor that works to its advantage is that everyone is interested, at one time or another, in finding out about the workings of his or her brain. Similarly, public concern about the social ills of substance abuse, a concern now as widespread as the afflictions themselves, could be the opening needed to convince the public of the importance of brain research for understanding and treating addictions.

A simple way to measure the health of a scientific discipline might be to ask a gathering of its practitioners, "Would you encourage your best young students to enter the field nowadays?" Allan Bromley, while traveling around the country and meeting with groups in many scientific fields, has found that the answer tends to be no, and the reason often given is that the particular field under discussion is not as much fun as it used to be.

For neuroscience, the answer was a little different. Some said no, just as many said yes, and perhaps the greatest number emphatically answered both yes and no. Surprisingly, a clear consensus emerged from all this: while the science itself is more exciting than ever and the practical applications of one's work may be most gratifying, finding subsistence in the field has become more and more difficult and time consuming, and the prospects are discouraging. A senior scientist may well hesitate before encouraging young investigators to enter the field—particularly if the funding prospects to sustain a career show no signs of improving and a scientist's time is increasingly taken up with the search for funds rather than with research. The long-time chairman of one neurology department put the matter succinctly: "The doing is sensational now. It's the not doing that's agony."

Huda Akil, of the Mental Health Research Institute at the University of Michigan, suggests that research groups or "teams" may offer young researchers some protection against too-early exposure to the fierce struggle for funds. With a senior scientist navigating the grant application process, young researchers are free to concentrate on their work. Although in no way a long-term solution to constraints in funding, the team approach offers at least partial shelter and makes use of the assurance and standing of researchers who have already spent some time in the field.

It is a simple but ironic sign of the times that neuroscience should be facing some of the greatest research challenges the field has ever seen just when it is becoming clear that there may no longer be the resources to tackle them as they deserve.

The knowledge gained from past decades coupled with today's powerful technologies for imaging, magnifying, assembling data, and cloning cells make for fascinating research possibilities; the means for translating research findings into therapeutic benefits are increasing all the time; but budgets have rarely been so tight. Public funds are being strained to the limit—and still the list of social ills continues to grow, increasing the competition for these strained resources.

In a society struggling with a weak domestic economy, a decline in public education, the deterioration of cities, and a staggering one-fifth of the population living in poverty, science must make the broadest possible case for what it can contribute toward healing these ills. Public support for brain research in the near future may depend on the success with which the scientific and health care communities, and other parties sympathetic to their aims, can convey the excitement, the fascination, and above all the public value of neuroscience. The time is right for building alliances between the public and private sectors that can bring the research agenda, talent, funding, and logistical support for these efforts all together. Neuroscience is poised for dazzling progress in the next 10 years.

ACKNOWLEDGMENTS

Chapter 9 is based on a panel discussion entitled, "In the Coming Decade: What Needs To Be Done? What Can Be Done?" The panelists were D. Allan Bromley, assistant to the President for science and technology; Pete V. Domenici, United States senator; Frederick K. Goodwin, administrator of the Alcohol, Drug Abuse, and Mental Health Administration (ADAMHA); Alberto Grignolo, president of FIDIA Pharmaceutical Corporation; Thomas W. Langfitt, president of the Pew Charitable Trusts; James O. Mason, assistant secretary for health in the Department of Health and Human Services; and David T. Mahoney, president of David Mahoney Ventures and chairman of the Dana Foundations.

Suggested Readings

Bloom, Floyd E., and Mark A. Randolph, eds., Institute of Medicine. 1990. *Funding Health Sciences Research: A Strategy to Restore Balance.* Washington, D.C.: National Academy Press. 255 pp.

The Brain: A Scientific American Book. 1979. San Francisco: W. H. Freeman. 149 pp.

Calder, Nigel. 1971. *The Mind of Man: An Investigation into Current Research on the Brain and Human Nature.* New York: Viking Press. 288 pp.

Carey, Joseph, ed. 1990. *Brain Facts: A Primer on the Brain and Nervous System.* Washington, D.C.: Society for Neuroscience. 31 pp.

Cline, Harvey E., William E. Lorensen, Ron Kikinis, and Ferenc Jolesz. 1990. Technical note. Three-dimensional segmentation of MR images of the head using probability and connectivity. *J. Comput. Assist. Tomogr.* 14:1037-1045.

Curtis, Helena. 1983. *Biology*, 4th ed. New York: Worth Publishers. 1,110 pp.

Gazzaniga, Michael S. 1988. *Mind Matters: How Mind and Brain Interact to Create Our Conscious Lives.* Boston: Houghton Mifflin. 244 pp.

Haines, Duane E. 1987. *Neuroanatomy: An Atlas of Structures, Sections, and Systems*, 2d ed. Baltimore: Urban & Schwarzenberg, Inc. 228 pp.

Kandel, Eric R., and James H. Schwartz, eds. 1981. *Principles of Neural Science.* New York: Elsevier North Holland. 731 pp.

Kiernan, John A. 1987. *Introduction to Human Neuroscience.* Philadelphia: J. B. Lippincott Company. 232 pp.

Klawans, Harold L. 1991. *Newton's Madness: Further Tales of Clinical Neurology.* New York: HarperPerennial. 218 pp.

Noonan, David. 1989. *Neuro-: Life on the Frontlines of Brain Surgery and Neurological Medicine.* New York: Ballantine Books. 220 pp.

Pechura, Constance M., and Joseph B. Martin, eds., Institute of Medicine. 1991. *Mapping the Brain and Its Functions.* Washington, D.C.: National Academy Press. 141 pp.

Restak, Richard M. 1984. *The Brain.* New York: Bantam Books. 371 pp.

Sacks, Oliver. 1987. *The Man Who Mistook His Wife for a Hat, and Other Clinical Tales.* New York: HarperPerennial. 243 pp.

Shelton, Mark L. 1989. *Working in a Very Small Place: The Making of a Neurosurgeon.* New York: Vintage Books. 315 pp.

United States Congress, Office of Technology Assessment. 1991. *Federally Funded Research: Decisions for a Decade.* OTA-SET-490. Washington, D.C.: Government Printing Office.

White House Office of Science and Technology Policy. 1991. *Maximizing Human Potential: Decade of the Brain 1990-2000.* Federal Coordinating Council for Science, Engineering and Technology, Committee on Life Sciences and Health, Subcommittee on Brain and Behavioral Sciences. Washington, D.C. 98 pp.

Acknowledgments

This book was triggered by the July 1990 symposium that was organized by the Institute of Medicine to initiate the Decade of the Brain. The speakers listed below participated in the meeting and graciously cooperated during the preparation of the book:

*Huda Akil, Mental Health Research Institute, University of Michigan, Ann Arbor

Duane Alexander, National Institute of Child Health and Human Development, National Institutes of Health, Bethesda, Maryland

Floyd E. Bloom, Department of Neuropharmacology, Scripps Clinic and Research Foundation, La Jolla, California

D. Allan Bromley, Executive Office of the President, Washington, D.C.

Barbara Bush, Washington, D.C.

Silvio Conte (deceased), United States House of Representatives, Washington, D.C.

**W. Maxwell Cowan, Howard Hughes Medical Institute, Bethesda, Maryland

Pete V. Domenici, United States Senate, Washington, D.C.

*Patricia Goldman-Rakic, Department of Neuroscience, Yale University School of Medicine, New Haven, Connecticut

Murray Goldstein, National Institute of Neurological Disorders and Stroke, National Institutes of Health, Bethesda, Maryland

Frederick K. Goodwin, Alcohol, Drug Abuse, and Mental Health Administration, Rockville, Maryland

Enoch Gordis, National Institute on Alcohol Abuse and Alcoholism, Alcohol, Drug Abuse, and Mental Health Administration, Rockville, Maryland

Alberto Grignolo, FIDIA Pharmaceuticals, Washington, D.C.

Roger Guillemin, Whittier Institute, La Jolla, California

David H. Hubel, Department of Neurobiology, Harvard University Medical School, Boston, Massachusetts

Lily Yeh Jan, Department of Physiology, University of California, San Francisco

Richard T. Johnson, Department of Neurology, Johns Hopkins University School of Medicine, Baltimore, Maryland

Lewis L. Judd, National Institute of Mental Health, Alcohol, Drug Abuse, and Mental Health Administration, Rockville, Maryland

Eric R. Kandel, Center for Neurobiology and Behavior, Columbia University, New York, New York

Carl Kupfer, National Eye Institute, National Institutes of Health, Bethesda, Maryland

Thomas W. Langfitt, The Glenmede Trust Company and The Pew Charitable Trusts, Philadelphia, Pennsylvania

Robert Lefkowitz, Duke University Medical Center, Durham, North Carolina

Alan I. Leshner, National Institute of Mental Health, Alcohol, Drug Abuse, and Mental Health Administration, Rockville, Maryland

David T. Mahoney, David Mahoney Ventures, New York, New York

Joseph B. Martin, School of Medicine, University of California, San Francisco

James O. Mason, Department of Health and Human Services, Washington, D.C.

Guy M. McKhann, Zanvyl Krieger Mind/Brain Institute, Johns Hopkins University, Baltimore, Maryland

Vernon B. Mountcastle, Department of Neuroscience, Johns Hopkins University School of Medicine, Baltimore, Maryland

Michael I. Posner, Department of Psychology, University of Oregon, Eugene

*Dominick P. Purpura, Albert Einstein College of Medicine, Bronx, New York

*Marcus E. Raichle, Washington University School of Medicine, St. Louis, Missouri

Pasko Rakic, Section of Neuroanatomy, Yale University School of Medicine, New Haven, Connecticut

*Lewis P. Rowland, Department of Neurology, College of Physicians & Surgeons, Columbia University, New York, New York

Charles R. Schuster, National Institute on Drug Abuse, Alcohol, Drug Abuse, and Mental Health Administration, Rockville, Maryland

Terrence J. Sejnowski, Computational Neurobiology Laboratory, Salk Institute, San Diego, California

*Solomon H. Snyder, Department of Neuroscience, Johns Hopkins University School of Medicine, Baltimore, Maryland

Louis W. Sullivan, Department of Health and Human Services, Washington, D.C.

James D. Watson, Cold Spring Harbor Laboratory, Cold Spring Harbor, New York

T. Franklin Williams, National Institute on Aging, National Institutes of Health, Bethesda, Maryland

*Member, Steering Committee
**Chair, Steering Committee

Proclamation

PROCLAMATIONS
No. 6158

Proclamation 6158 of July 17, 1990

Decade of the Brain, 1990-1999

55 F.R. 29553

By the President of the United States of America

A Proclamation

The human brain, a 3-pound mass of interwoven nerve cells that controls our activity, is one of the most magnificent—and mysterious—wonders of creation. The seat of human intelligence, interpreter of senses, and controller of movement, this incredible organ continues to intrigue scientist and layman alike.

Over the years, our understanding of the brain—how it works, what goes wrong when it is injured or diseased—has increased dramatically. However, we still have much more to learn. The need for continued study of the brain is compelling: millions of Americans are affected each year by disorders of the brain ranging from neurogenetic diseases to degenerative disorders such as Alzheimer's, as well as stroke, schizophrenia, autism, and impairments of speech, language, and hearing.

Today, these individuals and their families are justifiably hopeful, for a new era of discovery is dawning in brain research. Powerful microscopes, major strides in the study of genetics, and advanced brain imaging devices are giving physicians and scientists ever greater insight into the brain. Neuroscientists are mapping the brain's biochemical circuitry, which may help produce more effective drugs for alleviating the suffering of those who have Alzheimer's or Parkinson's disease. By studying how the brain's cells and chemicals develop, interact, and communicate with the rest of the body, investigators are also developing improved treatments for people incapacitated by spinal cord injuries, depressive disorders, and epileptic seizures. Breakthroughs in molecular genetics show great promise of yielding methods to treat and prevent Huntington's disease, the muscular dystrophies, and other life-threatening disorders.

Research may also prove valuable in our war on drugs, as studies provide greater insight into how people become addicted to drugs and how drugs affect the brain. These studies may also help produce effective treatments for chemical dependency and help us to understand and prevent the harm done to the preborn children of pregnant women who abuse drugs and alcohol. Because there is a connection between the body's nervous and immune systems, studies of the brain may also help enhance our understanding of Acquired Immune Deficiency Syndrome.

Many studies regarding the human brain have been planned and conducted by scientists at the National Institutes of Health, the National Institute of Mental Health, and other Federal research agencies. Augmenting Federal efforts are programs supported by private foundations and industry. The cooperation between these agencies and the multidisciplinary efforts of thousands of scientists and health care professionals provide powerful evidence of our Nation's determination to conquer brain disease.

To enhance public awareness of the benefits to be derived from brain research, the Congress, by House Joint Resolution 174, has designated the

PROCLAMATIONS
No. 6159

decade beginning January 1, 1990, as the "Decade of the Brain" and has authorized and requested the President to issue a proclamation in observance of this occasion.

NOW, THEREFORE, I, GEORGE BUSH, President of the United States of America, do hereby proclaim the decade beginning January 1, 1990, as the Decade of the Brain. I call upon all public officials and the people of the United States to observe that decade with appropriate programs, ceremonies, and activities.

IN WITNESS WHEREOF, I have hereunto set my hand this seventeenth day of July, in the year of our Lord nineteen hundred and ninety, and of the Independence of the United States of America the two hundred and fifteenth.

George Bush

Index

169

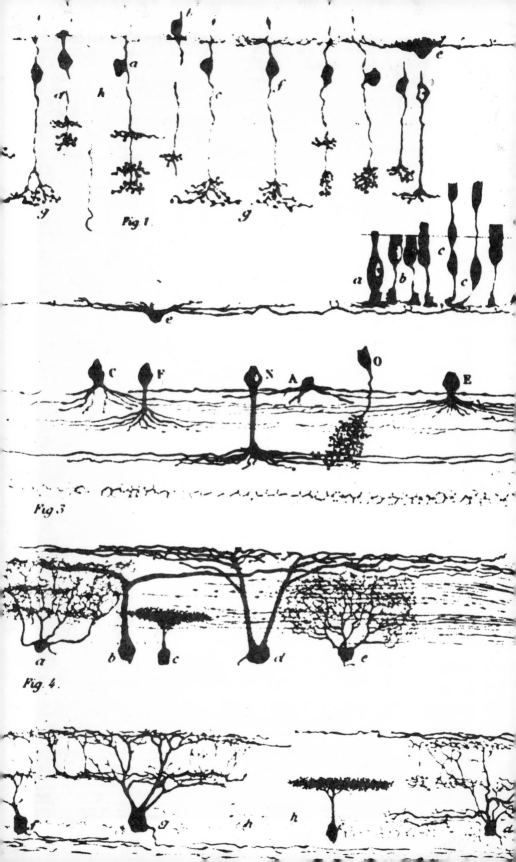

Fig 1.

Fig 3.

Fig. 4.